ABNORMAL MINDS

INDEX To The NEUROCOGNITIVE DISORDERS

ABSTRACT

With today's clinicians under such duress to practice evidence-based medicine in the most economical time frame, an Artificial-Intelligence-System assistance becomes compulsory. This Index to the Neurocognitive Disorders is the foundation of one such system designed to make accurate and rapid neurocognitive assessments possible. Yet there is no substitution for fact-checking which is the personal responsibility of each clinician - - - not of this manual.

JAMES PAUL BENVENUTI, M.D.

ABNORMAL MINDS

An individual who purchases this manual is allowed to reproduce copyrighted portions - for individual practice and may even convert to electronic recordings but only for the individual's clinical practice - unless permission is obtained from the copyright holder.

This book is dedicated to All Students seeking an easier understanding of the Neurocognitive Diagnoses.

Copyright © 2020, 2021, 2022

James Paul Benvenuti, M.D.

ISBN 9781387728466

About the Author

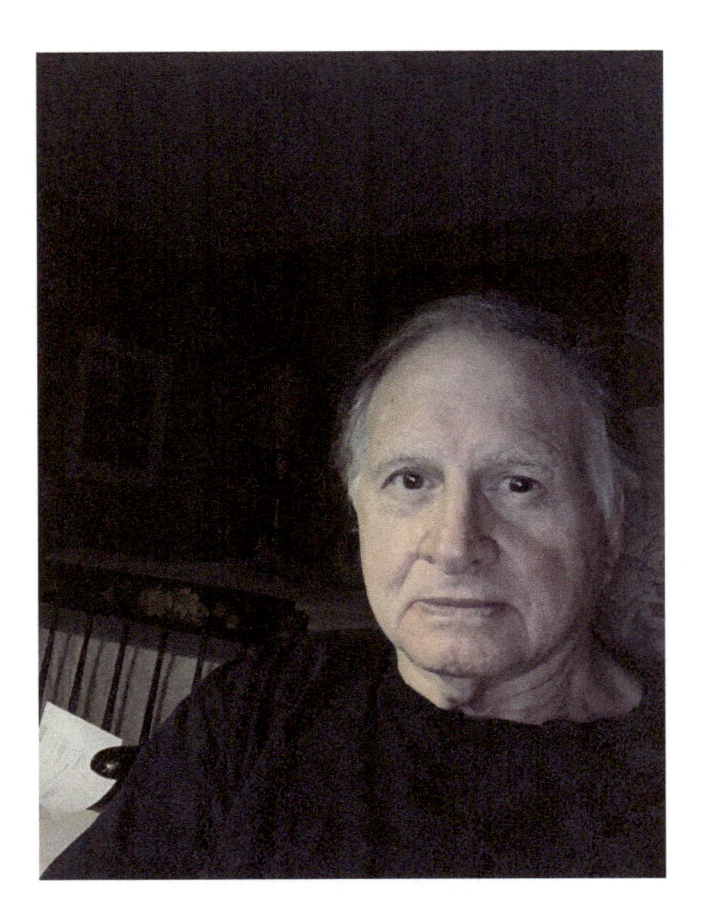

Doctor James Paul Benvenuti, M.D. is a board-certified pediatrician who completed a fellowship in Pediatric Psychoneurology at U.C.S.F. Medical Center, studied neurology at U.C.L.A. Medical Center and Adult Psychiatry at the Walter Reed Army Medical Center. For 20 years he was the staff psychiatrist at the Glen Roberts Child Study Center working with the developer of the Roberts-2 analytical assessment of emotionality and cognition. Doctor Benvenuti published "NORMAL MINDS" in 2016. He then wrote this document after utilizing it on hundreds of Mental Status Examinations.

TABLE OF CONTENTS

Page TITLE

- 5 Introduction
- 10 Ch. 1a: The NeuroDiagnostic Questionnaire
- 27 Ch. 1b. DIAGOSTICS
- 41 Ch. 2 Health History/ R.O.S.
- 73 Ch. 3 EXAMINATIONS
- 98 Ch. 4 DELIRIUM
- 127 Ch. 5 AMNESTIC DISORDERS
- 134 Ch. 6 DEMENTIA & NCDs
- 153 INDEX to the NeuroCognitive Disorders
- 165 References

INTRODUCTION

Although the categories for the Neurocognitive Disorders in the 5th Edition of the American Psychiatric Association's **Diagnostic And Statistical Manual Of Mental Disorders** appear simple (limited to *Delirium, Amnestic Disorders, and Dementia)*, their "Major and Mild Neurocognitive Disorders Due To Another Medical Condition" and "… Due to Multiple Etiologies", or "Due to Unspecified Neurocognitive Disorder" categories present a differential diagnostic challenge which is daunting. And treatment is precarious without specification of etiology. DSM-5 discusses only 15 of such etiologies. This" INDEX To The Neurocognitive Disorders" guides the clinician to more than 200 etiologies with their supportive Algorithms. It was developed to assist the clinician in approaching the complaints of patients and their caregivers with a logical and methodical "lock-step" system of assessment. These will be primarily complaints of *deterioration* in:

ABSTRACT THINKING: categorization/ conceptualization/ creativity; SPEECH & Language.

AFFECT: feelings / mood.

ATTENTION: focus/ concentration/ persistence / processing speed and overcoming distractibility.

BEHAVIOR: personality changes / "acting strange"

DRIVE: ambition/ energy/ "drive".

FUNCTIONAL CAPACITIES: milestones/ work performance/ capacity for performing Activities of Daily Living and capacity to **maintain** relationships with others.

INSIGHT: self-appraisals of cognitive functioning / feelings/ motives / intentions / problems.

JUDGMENT: mores/ morals/ intelligent choices.

MEMORY: immediate/ intermediate/ remote.

ORIENTATION: to time / place/ person or circumstances.

This deterioration of capacities (which had been previously acquired) may nevertheless have a **genetic** etiology and therefore may also have a **variable** age of onset.

The Neurocognitive Questionnaire of **CHAPTER 1a** is an amalgamation of field-tested, statistically documented psychological scales designed to screen for specific neurocognitive categories. These are either in the public domain or are printed after requesting permission from the copyright holders. The **sorted version** which follows in **CHAPTER 1b** may be utilized by the clinician to screen for specific problems, such as:

(1) **ANXIETY DISORDERS**;

(2) **AUTISM SPECTRUM DISORDERS** which sometimes can be confused with incipient schizophrenia;

(3) **BIPOLAR DISORDER; MANIC STATE** (which is often confused with "delirium");

(4) **DELIRIUM:** an abrupt onset of a confusional state.

(5) **DEMENTIA** (with its 7 stages);

(6) **MAJOR DEPRESSIVE DISORDER** (which can confound the clinician who doesn't consider "pseudodementia" of depression;

(7) **SLEEP DISORDERS** (which can sometimes seem to be a delirium);

(8) **VERY FUNCTIONALLY IMPAIRED:** which must be distinguished from **physically** impaired; and the two can coexist.

CHAPTER 2 is a Health History which functions as a Review of Systems to screen for the multiple medical disorders which can cause more than 200 of the Neurocognitive Disorders Due To Another Medical Condition. These may be printed or utilized in a computer-assisted screening system to accelerate the diagnostic process. The patient or caregiver is responsible for compiling a history of complaints but always it is the clinician who must function as the **"fact-checker"**. And the major responsibility of the clinician (within the limited time available) is to perform a meticulous **Mental Status Examination** which can be found in **CHAPTER 3.** All of this data can then be categorized by utilizing the **Mental Status Examination Summary Sheet** located at the end of **CHAPTER 3.**

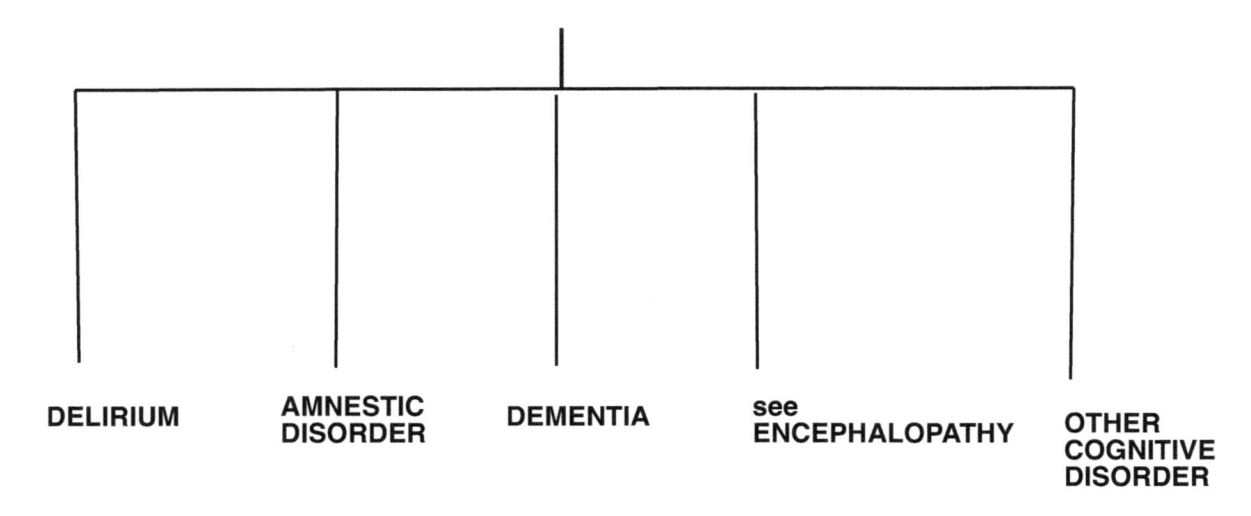

NEUROCOGNITIVE DISORDERS
are deterioration in a person's ATTENTION; MEMORY; LEARNED SOCIAL MORES or BEHAVIORS: this implies deterioration in what was PREVIOUSLY ACQUIRED. THEY MAY, NEVERTHELESS, HAVE A CONGENITAL OR GENETIC CAUSE WHICH HAS A VARIABLE ONSET.

- **DELIRIUM**
- **AMNESTIC DISORDER**
- **DEMENTIA**
- see **ENCEPHALOPATHY**
- **OTHER COGNITIVE DISORDER**

Ch 1a. The NeuroCognitive Questionnaire

PLEASE ANSWER THESE QUESTIONS AS BEST AS YOU CAN BY PLACING AN "X" IN THE PROPER COLUMN FOR "NEVER"; "SOMETIMES"; "OFTEN" OR "VERY OFTEN"

NEVER	SOMETIMES	OFTEN	Very Often	COMPLAINT
				I HAVE BEEN GETTING SO FORGETFUL, I HAVE DIFFICULTY FINDING THE RIGHT WORD & PEOPLES NAMES.
				I CAN FEEL MY HEART BEATING FAST.
				I'VE BEEN VERY NERVOUS AND I'VE EVEN GOTTEN VIOLENT AT TIMES.
				I GET FEELINGS OF NUMBNESS AND TINGLING IN MY FINGERS, TOES.
				I CAN WORK AT ASSISTED LIVING.
				IT IS DIFFICULT FOR ME TO WORK AND FUNCTION IN GROUPS.
				I FEEL WEAK AND GET TIRED EASILY.
				I HAVE HAD IDEAS ABOUT KILLING MYSELF.
				I HAVE TO HAVE HELP FEEDING MYSELF AND GOING TO THE TOILET.
				I CAN INITIATE A CONVERSATION WITH FRIENDS.
				I CAN FALL ASLEEP AS A PASSENGER IN A CAR FOR AN HOUR WITHOUT A BREAK.
				I CAN CHAT AND MAKE SMALL TALK WITH PEOPLE.

NEVER	SOMETIMES	OFTEN	Very Often	**COMPLAINT**
				I CAN BALANCE A CHECKBOOK.
				I AM VERY DISTRACTIBLE.
				I DREAMED ABOUT KILLING MYSELF.
				I AM BOTHERED BY STOMACH ACHES OR INDIGESTION.
				I HAVE WISHED I WERE DEAD.
				I USUALLY FEEL SO SAD MUCH OF THE TIME.
				MY ARMS AND LEGS SHAKE AND TREMBLE.
				AT TIMES I DID "UNUSUAL" THINGS - FOOLISH OR RISKY OR EXCESSIVE THINGS ACCORDING TO OTHERS.
				WHEN TALKING TO SOMEONE, I HAVE A HARD TIME TELLING WHEN IT IS MY TURN TO TALK OR TO LISTEN.
				VERY SUDDENLY I HAVE SPELLS OF POOR JUDGMENT/ MEMORY PROBLEMS/ SLOWED THINKING OR SPEECH.
				SOMETIMES I HAVE TO COVER MY EARS TO BLOCK OUT PAINFUL NOISES (like people talking too much or too loudly).
				THEY SAY I'M CRAZY" BECAUSE I "SEE THINGS" - THAT OTHERS DON'T SEE.
				AT TIMES I HAVE FELT MUCH MORE SELF-CONFIDENT THAN USUAL.
				I HAVE MUCH TROUBLE WALKING PROPERLY NOW.

NEVER	SOMETIMES	OFTEN	Very Often	**COMPLAINT**
				I HAVE BEEN FORGETTING HOW TO DRESS MYSELF CORRECTLY.
				WHEN I START A PROJECT I REALLY DON'T EXPECT TO SUCCEED WITH IT.
				I HAVE TO EMPTY MY BLADDER OFTEN.
				I HAVE BEEN IN HIGH PLACES AND FELT LIKE JUMPING.
				I HAVE DIFFICULTY CONCENTRATING FOR EXTENDED PERIODS OF TIME.
				I HAVE BEEN GETTING SO FORGETFUL, I GET LOST WHEN TRAVELING IN UNFAMILIAR LOCATIONS.
				I'M NOT SURE THE PERSON LIVING WITH ME IS REALLY MY SPOUSE - IT DOESN'T SEEM POSSIBLE.
				MY SLEEP PATTERNS ARE SO DISTURBED NOW.
				I HAVE BEEN HAVING PROBLEMS KNOWING HOW TO TRAVEL ALONE NOW - I NEED SOMEONE WITH ME.
				I HAVE DIFFICULTY CARRYING OUT COMPLEX INSTRUCTIONS.
				I HAVE NEGLECTED MY FAMILY BECAUSE OF MY USE OF ILLEGAL DRUGS.
				I FEEL HOPEFUL ABOUT THE FUTURE.
				I PREFER TO WIN RATHER THAN LOSE WHEN I PLAY GAMES.
				MY LIFE PARTNER (OR PARENTS) HAVE COMPLAINED ABOUT MY INVOLVEMENT WITH DRUGS.

NEVER	SOMETIMES	OFTEN	Very Often	**COMPLAINT**
				I HAVE BEEN GETTING SO FORGETFUL OF OTHER PEOPLE'S NAMES.
				I HAVE BEEN GETTING CONFUSED TRYING TO BE ON TIME AND GETTING TO THE RIGHT PLACE.
				MY HANDS ARE USUALLY COLD AND "CLAMMY".
				I FALL ASLEEP EASILY AND GET A GOOD NIGHT'S REST.
				I AM NOT HAPPY WITH MY SEX LIFE.
				I CAN WORK WITH COMPUTERS.
				I'VE LOST THE ABILITY TO "HOLD MY URINE" NOW.
				I CAN FALL ASLEEP JUST WATCHING TELEVISION.
				I CAN BREATHE IN AND OUT EASILY.
				I HAVE BEEN GETTING SO FORGETFUL, MY WORK IS STARTING TO SUFFER.
				I HAVE DIFFICULTY PRONOUNCING WORDS CLEARLY SO OTHERS CAN UNDERSTAND ME.
				AT TIMES I FELT SO GOOD OR "HYPER" THAT I EVEN GOT INTO TROUBLE.
				VERY SUDDENLY I CAN GET CONFUSIONAL SPELLS.
				I NOTICE THAT I AM LOSING WEIGHT.

NEVER	SOMETIMES	OFTEN	Very Often	**COMPLAINT**
				I HAVE USED DRUGS OTHER THAN THOSE REQUIRED FOR MEDICAL REASONS.
				I HAVE GOTTEN SO DISCOURAGED THAT I THOUGHT ABOUT ENDING MY LIFE.
				I HAVE DIFFICULTY PLANNING AND ORGANIZING THINGS.
				I HAVE CRYING SPELLS OR FEEL LIKE IT OFTEN.
				I AM MORE IRRITABLE THAN USUAL.
				MY LIFE SEEMS SO EMPTY.
				I HAVE A CURRENT DRIVER'S LICENSE.
				I HAVE FELT LIKE RUNNING INTO TRAFFIC.
				WHEN I AM BY MYSELF, I FEEL THE HAPPIEST.
				MY FACE GETS HOT AND BLUSHES.
				I CAN CORRECTLY PAY THE BILLS.
				I FEEL CALM AND CAN SIT STILL EASILY.
				I DO REMEMBER A LITTLE BIT ABOUT MY PAST LIFE.
				I CAN'T EVEN CONVERSE WITH THE FAMILY IF THE TELEVISION OR OTHERS ARE DISTRACTING ME NEARBY.

NEVER	SOMETIMES	OFTEN	Very Often	**COMPLAINT**
				I CAN SHOWER AND BATHE BY MYSELF.
				I CAN COOK A WHOLE MEAL BY MYSELF.
				IT IS DIFFICULT FOR ME TO UNDERSTAND HOW OTHER PEOPLE ARE FEELING WHEN WE ARE TALKING.
				AT TIMES I WAS MUCH MORE SOCIAL/ OUTGOING THAN USUAL (like TELEPHONING FRIENDS IN THE MIDDLE OF THE NIGHT).
				AT TIMES I WAS MUCH MORE INTERESTED IN SEX THAN USUAL.
				MY HEART BEATS FASTER THAN USUAL.
				I FEEL THAT OTHERS WOULD BE BETTER OFF IF I WERE DEAD.
				I FOCUS ON DETAILS RATHER THAN THE OVERALL IDEA.
				I GET UPSET EASILY OR FEEL PANICKY.
				I HAD A PLAN OF HOW I WOULD KILL MYSELF.
				THEY SAY I'M CRAZY" BECAUSE I "SEE THINGS" - (LIGHTS & COLORS) THAT OTHERS DON'T SEE.
				I HAVE BEEN GETTING SO FORGETFUL PEOPLE SAY - BUT I JUST DON'T BELIEVE IT.
				I CAN FALL ASLEEP JUST SITTING QUIETLY AFTER A LUNCH WITHOUT ALCOHOL.
				I HAVE BEEN HAVING PROBLEMS TRYING TO DO THINGS WITHOUT HELP FROM OTHERS.

NEVER	SOMETIMES	OFTEN	Very Often	**COMPLAINT**

I CAN WALK FAR FROM HOME

I EVEN NEED ASSISTANCE FEEDING MYSELF AND WITH MY TOILET NEEDS.

I CAN CLEAN THE WHOLE HOUSE.

I'VE LOST THE ABILITY TO COMMUNICATE NOW.

I HAVE TROUBLE SLEEPING THROUGH THE NIGHT.

AT TIMES I WAS MUCH MORE ACTIVE OR "DID MORE THINGS" THAN USUAL.

I STILL ENJOY THE THINGS I USED TO.

THEY SAY I'M SHOWING "NEUROLOGICAL SIGNS" NOW.

I HAVE HAD MEDICAL PROBLEMS AS A RESULT OF MY DRUG USE (e.g., MEMORY LOSS/ HEPATITIS/ CONVULSIONS, ETC.)

I DON'T FEEL THAT I AM USEFUL OR NEEDED.

AT TIMES I HAVE SENSED MY SOUL LEAVING MY BODY.

AT TIMES I HAD MUCH MORE ENERGY THAN USUAL.

AT TIMES I FELT SO GOOD OR "HYPER" THAT OTHERS THOUGHT I WAS "NOT MY NORMAL SELF

NEVER	SOMETIMES	OFTEN	Very Often	COMPLAINT
				I TAKE THINGS TOO LITERALLY, SO I OFTEN MISS WHAT PEOPLE ARE TRYING TO SAY.
				I HAVE TROUBLE WITH CONSTIPATION.
				I HAVE BEEN GETTING SO FORGETFUL, MY HOME LIFE IS STARTING TO SUFFER.
				SOME ORDINARY TEXTURES THAT DO NOT BOTHER OTHERS FEEL VERY OFFENSIVE WHEN THEY TOUCH MY SKIN.
				I HAVE THOUGHT ABOUT WAYS TO KILL MYSELF.
				I CAN GET OUT OF BED ON TIME.
				I HAVE NIGHTMARES.
				I HAVE HAD BLACKOUTS OR FLASHBACKS AS A RESULT OF DRUG USE.
				I HAVE DRUNK ALCOHOLIC BEVERAGES.
				I HAVE EPISODES WHERE PEOPLE CAN'T UNDERSTAND WHAT I AM TRYING TO SAY.
				I HAVE BEEN HAVING PROBLEMS AT WORK AND HOME BECAUSE I'M FORGETTING WHAT'S IN THE NEWS.
				I HAVE BEEN HAVING PROBLEMS AT WORK AND HOME BECAUSE OF MY MEMORY.
				I FEEL THAT EVERYTHING IS ALL RIGHT AND NOTHING BAD WILL HAPPEN.
				I GET TIRED FOR NO REASON.

NEVER	SOMETIMES	OFTEN	Very Often	COMPLAINT
				I FEEL AFRAID FOR NO REASON AT ALL
				I DON'T PAY ATTENTION TO WHAT SEASON IT IS OR WHAT HOLIDAY IS "COMING UP".
				AT TIMES I WAS MUCH MORE TALKATIVE AND SPOKE MUCH FASTER THAN USUAL.
				I FIND IT EASY TO MAKE DECISIONS.
				A HEALTH PROFESSIONAL HAS TOLD ME I WAS "BIPOLAR" OR "MANIC-DEPRESSIVE.
				I HAVE DIFFICULTY FOLLOWING THROUGH AND "FINISHING" PROJECTS.
				I HAVE DIFFICULTY CONCENTRATING.
				I HAVE EXPERIENCED MUCH NAUSEA AND VOMITING LATELY.
				I HAVE ENGAGED IN ILLEGAL ACTIVITIES IN ORDER TO OBTAIN DRUGS.
				I HAVE BEEN GETTING SO FORGETFUL, I HAVE BEEN LOSING THINGS.
				I'VE LOST ALL MY "DRIVE" - I JUST DON'T CARE ABOUT ANYTHING ANYMORE.
				IT IS DIFFICULT TO FIGURE OUT WHAT OTHER PEOPLE EXPECT OF ME.
				SOMETIMES I HAVE TO COVER MY EARS TO BLOCK OUT PAINFUL NOISES (LIKE THE VACUUM CLEANERS).
				I CAN TAKE THE BUS BY MYSELF.

NEVER	SOMETIMES	OFTEN	Very Often	**COMPLAINT**
				I FEEL LIKE I'M FALLING APART AND "GOING TO PIECES".
				I CAN CARE ABOUT OTHERS.
				I DON'T REMEMBER WHAT'S HAPPENING IN THE NEWS OR EVEN IN MY OWN FAMILY.
				AT TIMES I WAS SO IRRITABLE I SHOUTED AT PEOPLE OR STARTED ARGUMENTS OR FIGHTS.
				I ENJOY LOOKING AT, TALKING TO AND BEING WITH ATTRACTIVE WOMEN/MEN.
				I CANNOT FOCUS ON A SUBJECT VERY WELL.
				I CAN WATCH TV AND REMEMBER MUCH.
				I HAVE THOUGHT ABOUT KILLING MYSELF BUT DID NOT TRY TO DO IT.
				I CAN MAKE CORRECT CHANGE.
				I HAVE BLOOD RELATIVES DIAGNOSED AS "BIPOLAR" OR "MANIC-DEPRESSIVE"1
				I EAT AS MUCH AS I USED TO.
				I CAN SHOP IN THE STORES FOR MY CLOTHES.
				I HAVE FAINTING SPELLS OR FEEL LIKE IT.
				MY MIND IS AS CLEAR AS IT USED TO BE.

NEVER	SOMETIMES	OFTEN	Very Often	**COMPLAINT**

I BELIEVE MY FATHER WAS AS GOOD A MAN AS HE COULD BE.

I CAN FEED MYSELF.

I CAN INITIATE A CONVERSATION WITH STRANGERS.

I HAVE SMOKED MARIJUANA.

I CAN FALL ASLEEP JUST SITTING AND TALKING TO SOMEONE.

I HAVE BEEN FORGETTING THE NAMES OF MY SPOUSE AND MY CHILDREN.

I AM UNABLE TO STOP USING DRUGS WHEN I WANT TO.

I FIND IT HARD TO DO THE THINGS I USED TO.

AT TIMES I WAS SO EASILY DISTRACTED BY THINGS AROUND ME, I HAD TROUBLE CONCENTRATING/ "STAYING ON TRACK".

I AM BOTHERED BY HEADACHES, NECK AND BACK PAINS.

THEY SAY I'LL CLEAN THE HOUSE ALL DAY OR RAKE LEAVES ALL AFTERNOON - REPETITIVELY.

THEY SAY I'M CRAZY" BECAUSE I "HEAR VOICES" SOMETIMES.

I OFTEN DON'T KNOW HOW TO ACT IN SOCIAL SITUATIONS.

THEY SAY I'M CRAZY" BECAUSE I SMELL "STRANGE SMELLS" SOMETIMES.

NEVER	SOMETIMES	OFTEN	Very Often	**COMPLAINT**
				AT TIMES THOUGHTS "RACED" THROUGH MY HEAD AND I COULDN'T SLOW MY THOUGHTS DOWN.
				I CAN DRIVE A CAR.
				ALMOST DAILY I THINK I WOULD BE BETTER OFF IF I WERE DEAD.
				I CAN SOLVE SOME DIFFICULT PROBLEMS.
				I HAVE BEEN HAVING PROBLEMS KNOWING HOW TO PAY MY BILLS NOW.
				IT CAN BE VERY HARD TO READ SOMEONE'S FACE, HAND, AND BODY MOVEMENTS WHEN WE ARE TALKING.
				WHEN I FEEL OVERWHELMED BY MY SENSES, I HAVE TO ISOLATE MYSELF TO SHUT THEM DOWN.
				VERY SUDDENLY I HAVE SPELLS OF CONFUSION ABOUT THE DATE OR "WHERE I AM".
				I FEEL MORE NERVOUS AND ANXIOUS THAN USUAL
				I HAVE BEEN HAVING PROBLEMS TAKING ON NEW ASSIGNMENTS - I FEAR FAILURE.
				I HAVE DREAMED ABOUT DEATH.
				I HAVE BEEN FORGETTING MY OWN NAME SOMETIMES.
				I CAN DISCUSS CURRENT EVENTS WITH FRIENDS.
				I HAVE BEEN HAVING PROBLEMS AT WORK AND HOME BECAUSE I CAN'T CONCENTRATE ANYMORE.

NEVER	SOMETIMES	OFTEN	Very Often	**COMPLAINT**
				I CAN USE CORRECT ENGLISH.
				I HAVE DIFFICULTY READING AND WRITING.
				I HAVE HAD MEDICAL PROBLEMS AS A RESULT OF MY DRUG USE (e.g., MEMORY LOSS/ HEPATITIS/ CONVULSIONS, ETC.)
				I HAVE BEEN GETTING SO FORGETFUL, IT IS MAKING ME SO "NERVOUS".
				I DON'T THINK ANYONE REALLY CARES WHAT HAPPENS TO ME.
				AT TIMES I HAD UNUSUALLY MORE ENERGY THAN ORDINARY.
				HOW TO MAKE FRIENDS AND SOCIALIZE IS A MYSTERY TO ME.
				I HAVE FELT LIKE LIFE WAS NOT WORTH LIVING.
				I HAVE DIFFICULTY THINKING CLEARLY AND EFFICIENTLY.
				ALL MY FOOD TASTES THE SAME.
				I AM ABLE TO STAY OVERNIGHT AT A FRIEND'S HOUSE.
				I HAVE USED ALCOHOL EXCESSIVELY.
				I CAN READ FROM A BOOK AND REMEMBER MUCH.
				I HAD A PLAN TO KILL MYSELF; STARTED TO DO IT & THEN STOPPED AT THE LAST MINUTE.

NEVER	SOMETIMES	OFTEN	Very Often	**COMPLAINT**
				I CAN WORK WITH TOOLS.
				I CAN FALL ASLEEP JUST SITTING AND READING.
				THEY SAY I'M CRAZY" BECAUSE I SUSPECT CONSPIRACIES THAT OTHERS DON'T UNDERSTAND.
				I CAN FALL ASLEEP LYING DOWN TO REST IN THE AFTERNOON WHEN CIRCUMSTANCES PERMIT.
				I HAVE HAD EPISODES OF "SLOWED THINKING" (WITHOUT ANY ALCOHOL OR DRUG USE).
				I AM BOTHERED BY DIZZY SPELLS.
				I CAN RIDE A BICYCLE.
				I TRIED TO KILL MYSLEF.
				I LIKE EVERYONE I KNOW.
				I HAVE BEEN HAVING PROBLEMS AT WORK AND HOME BECAUSE I'M FORGETTING PEOPLE'S BIRTHDAYS, ANNIVERSARIES, ETC.
				PEOPLE SAY MY "PERSONALITY" HAS CHANGED SO MUCH.
				I CAN FALL ASLEEP IN A CAR, WHILE STOPPED FOR A FEW MINUTES IN THE TRAFFIC.
				I HAVE BEEN GETTING SO FORGETFUL.
				I HAVE SMOKED CIGARETTES.

NEVER	SOMETIMES	OFTEN	Very Often	COMPLAINT
				I CAN'T EVEN WATCH TV IF THE FAMILY IS TALKING NEARBY.
				I HAVE USED MORE THAN ONE NON-PRESCRIBED DRUG AT A TIME.
				I GET EXTREMELY UPSET WHEN THE WAY I LIKE TO DO THINGS IS SUDDENLY CHANGED.
				I HAVE BEEN GETTING SO FORGETFUL OF APPOINTMENTS, FOR EXAMPLE WITH DOCTORS.
				SOMETIMES I GET ANGRY.
				I CAN'T MAKE DECISIONS ANYMORE - IT "TAKES TOO MUCH OUT OF ME".
				SOMETIMES I DO TELL LITTLE LIES.
				THERE HAVE BEEN FREQUENT ATTEMPTS TO ROB ME.
				I HAVE EXPERIENCED WITHDRAWL SYMPTOMS (FELT SICK) WHEN I STOPPED TAKING DRUGS.
				I CAN CLEAN THE YARD.
				I TALKED TO SOMEONE ABOUT KILLING MYSELF.
				I HAVE BEEN HAVING PROBLEMS GROWING OLD BUT I KNOW IT'S JUST NORMAL FOR MY AGE.
				I AM HYPERSENSITIVE TO LIGHT/ "GLARE".
				I HAVE TAKEN DRUGS OTHER THAN MARIJUANA OR PRESCRIPTION DRUGS.

NEVER	SOMETIMES	OFTEN	Very Often	**COMPLAINT**
				I HAVE THOUGHT ABOUT DEATH AND DYING.
				AT TIMES I GOT MUCH LESS SLEEP THAN USUAL & FOUND THAT I DIDN'T REALLY MISS IT.
				I AM ABLE TO LEAVE THE HOUSE ALONE.
				I HAVE BEEN GETTING SO FORGETFUL, I AM WORRIED ABOUT IT.
				I DON'T THINK MY SINS CAN BE FORGIVEN.
				I HAVE BEEN FORGETTING NAMES OF CLOSE FAMILY MEMBERS, TELEPHONE NUMBERS I ONCE KNEW & ADDRESSES.
				SOMETIMES I PERCEIVE THINGS THAT ARE SO DIFFERENT FROM WHAT OTHER'S ARE SEEING.
				LAW ENFORCEMENT IS ONE OF MY IMPORTANT VALUES.
				I CAN DO THE DISHES.
				I HAVE BEEN GETTING SO FORGETFUL, I REMEMBER LITTLE I READ FROM A PAGE.
				I CAN READ FROM A BOOK.
				I AM ABLE TO VISIT A FRIEND WHEN I WANT TO.
				I CAN CLEAN MY ROOMS.
				I AM RESTLESS AND CAN'T KEEP STILL.

Ch. 1b: DIAGNOSTICS

AUTISM SPECTRUM DISORDERS

ASPERGER.....ASSESSMENT

CLIENT:
DATE:

DETERMINE TO WHAT DEGREE .... THESE QUALITIES ARE PRESENT

	Some	Much More	Very Much
SHOWS DIFFICULTY INITIATING & MAINTAINING EYE CONTACT	☐	☐	☐
SHOWS STRONG FOOD PREFERENCES & AVERSIONS	☐	☐	☐
SHOWS SELF-STIMULATORY BEHAVIOR TO REDUCE ANXIETY	☐	☐	☐
SHOWS HIGH DISTRACTIBILITY WHEN ASKED TO ATTEND	☐	☐	☐
HAS COMPELLING NEED TO FINISH ONE TASK PRIOR TO CHANGING	☐	☐	☐
HAS DIFFICULTY STARTING A NEW PROJECT	☐	☐	☐
LOW MOTIVATION TO PERFORM TASK OF LITTLE PERSONAL INTEREST	☐	☐	☐
SHOWS RIGID ADHERENCE TO RULES & ROUTINES	☐	☐	☐
UNCOMFORTABLE COMPETING; CATASTROPHIC REACTION TO LOSS	☐	☐	☐
MUCH HIDDEN ANGER TOWARDS SELF & OTHERS; RESENTMENT	☐	☐	☐
DIFFICULTY EXPRESSING ANGER: "BOTTLING UP" ANGER	☐	☐	☐
OVERLOAD/MULTITASKING & CONTRADICTION CAUSES "SHUT-DOWN"	☐	☐	☐
SHOWS SARCASM, NEGATIVITY & CRITICISM	☐	☐	☐
GENERAL DIFFICULTY EXPRESSING MOST EMOTIONS	☐	☐	☐
GENERAL DIFFICULTY "READING" OTHER'S EMOTIONS	☐	☐	☐
PREFERS VISUALLY PRESENTED INSTRUCTIONS	☐	☐	☐

Notes:

	NEVER	SOMETIMES	OFTEN	Very Often	**COMPLAINT**
ANZIETY - ZUNG					MY HEART BEATS FASTER THAN USUAL.
ANXIETY - ZUNG					I FEEL MORE NERVOUS AND ANXIOUS THAN USUAL
ANXIETY - ZUNG					I FEEL AFRAID FOR NO REASON AT ALL
ANXIETY - ZUNG					I GET UPSET EASILY OR FEEL PANICKY.
ANXIETY - ZUNG					I FEEL LIKE I'M FALLING APART AND "GOING TO PIECES".
ANXIETY - ZUNG					I FEEL THAT EVERYTHING IS ALL RIGHT AND NOTHING BAD WILL HAPPEN.
ANXIETY - ZUNG					MY ARMS AND LEGS SHAKE AND TREMBLE.
ANXIETY - ZUNG					I AM BOTHERED BY HEADACHES, NECK AND BACK PAINS.
ANXIETY - ZUNG					I FEEL WEAK AND GET TIRED EASILY.
ANXIETY - ZUNG	X				I FEEL CALM AND CAN SIT STILL EASILY.
ANXIETY - ZUNG					I CAN FEEL MY HEART BEATING FAST.
ANXIETY - ZUNG					I AM BOTHERED BY DIZZY SPELLS.
ANXIETY - ZUNG					I HAVE FAINTING SPELLS OR FEEL LIKE IT.
ANXIETY - ZUNG	X				I CAN BREATHE IN AND OUT EASILY.
ANXIETY - ZUNG					I GET FEELINGS OF NUMBNESS AND TINGLING IN MY FINGERS, TOES.
ANXIETY - ZUNG					I AM BOTHERED BY STOMACH ACHES OR INDIGESTION.
ANXIETY - ZUNG					I HAVE TO EMPTY MY BLADDER OFTEN.
ANXIETY - ZUNG					MY HANDS ARE USUALLY COLD AND "CLAMMY".
ANXIETY - ZUNG					MY FACE GETS HOT AND BLUSHES.
ANXIETY - ZUNG	X				I FALL ASLEEP EASILY AND GET A GOOD NIGHT'S REST.
ANXIETY - ZUNG					I HAVE NIGHTMARES.
ASPERGER ASSESSMENT p.28					WHEN TALKING TO SOMEONE, I HAVE A HARD TIME TELLING WHEN IT IS MY TURN TO TALK OR TO LISTEN.
ASPERGER ASSESSMENT p.28					SOMETIMES I HAVE TO COVER MY EARS TO BLOCK OUT PAINFUL NOISES (LIKE THE VACUUM CLEANERS).
ASPERGER ASSESSMENT p.28					IT IS DIFFICULT FOR ME TO UNDERSTAND HOW OTHER PEOPLE ARE FEELING WHEN WE ARE TALKING.
ASPERGER ASSESSMENT p.28					SOMETIMES I HAVE TO COVER MY EARS TO BLOCK OUT PAINFUL NOISES (like people talking too much or too
ASPERGER ASSESSMENT p.28					SOME ORDINARY TEXTURES THAT DO NOT BOTHER OTHERS FEEL VERY OFFENSIVE WHEN THEY TOUCH
ASPERGER ASSESSMENT p.28					IT CAN BE VERY HARD TO READ SOMEONE'S FACE, HAND, AND BODY MOVEMENTS WHEN WE ARE

ASPERGER ASSESSMENT p.28		IT IS DIFFICULT FOR ME TO WORK AND FUNCTION IN GROUPS.
ASPERGER ASSESSMENT p.28		I FOCUS ON DETAILS RATHER THAN THE OVERALL IDEA.
ASPERGER ASSESSMENT p.28		IT IS DIFFICULT TO FIGURE OUT WHAT OTHER PEOPLE EXPECT OF ME.
ASPERGER ASSESSMENT p.28		I TAKE THINGS TOO LITERALLY, SO I OFTEN MISS WHAT PEOPLE ARE TRYING TO SAY.
ASPERGER ASSESSMENT p.28		I OFTEN DON'T KNOW HOW TO ACT IN SOCIAL SITUATIONS.
ASPERGER ASSESSMENT p.28		I GET EXTREMELY UPSET WHEN THE WAY I LIKE TO DO THINGS IS SUDDENLY CHANGED.
ASPERGER ASSESSMENT p.28	X	I CAN CHAT AND MAKE SMALL TALK WITH PEOPLE.
ASPERGER ASSESSMENT p.28		WHEN I FEEL OVERWHELMED BY MY SENSES, I HAVE TO ISOLATE MYSELF TO SHUT THEM DOWN.
ASPERGER ASSESSMENT p.28		HOW TO MAKE FRIENDS AND SOCIALIZE IS A MYSTERY TO ME.
ATYPICAL (T) ROBERTS-2 VERY OFTEN		I DON'T THINK MY SINS CAN BE FORGIVEN.
ATYPICAL (T) ROBERTS-2 VERY OFTEN		ALL MY FOOD TASTES THE SAME.
ATYPICAL (T) ROBERTS-2 VERY OFTEN		I DON'T THINK ANYONE REALLY CARES WHAT HAPPENS TO ME.
ATYPICAL (T) ROBERTS-2 VERY OFTEN		WHEN I AM BY MYSELF, I FEEL THE HAPPIEST.
ATYPICAL (F) ROBERTS-2 NEVER		LAW ENFORCEMENT IS ONE OF MY IMPORTANT VALUES.
ATYPICAL (T) ROBERTS-2 VERY OFTEN		WHEN I START A PROJECT I REALLY DON'T EXPECT TO SUCCEED WITH IT.
ATYPCIAL (T) ROBERTS-2 VERY OFTEN		I HAVE EXPERIENCED MUCH NAUSEA AND VOMITING LATELY.
ATYPICAL (T) ROBERTS-2 VERY OFTEN		AT TIMES I HAVE SENSED MY SOUL LEAVING MY BODY.
ATYPICAL (T) ROBERTS-2 VERY OFTEN		I AM NOT HAPPY WITH MY SEX LIFE.
ATYPICAL (T) ROBERTS-2 VERY OFTEN		THERE HAVE BEEN FREQUENT ATTEMPTS TO ROB ME.
ATYPICAL (F) ROBERTS-2 NEVER		I BELIEVE MY FATHER WAS AS GOOD A MAN AS HE COULD BE.

BIPOLAR - Mood Disorder Questionnaire	AT TIMES I WAS SO IRRITABLE I SHOUTED AT PEOPLE OR STARTED ARGUMENTS OR FIGHTS.
BIPOLAR - Mood Disorder Questionnaire	AT TIMES I GOT MUCH LESS SLEEP THAN USUAL & FOUND THAT I DIDN'T REALLY MISS IT.
BIPOLAR - Mood Disorder Questionnaire	AT TIMES I WAS MUCH MORE TALKATIVE AND SPOKE MUCH FASTER THAN USUAL.
BIPOLAR - Mood Disorder Questionnaire	AT TIMES THOUGHTS "RACED" THROUGH MY HEAD AND I COULDN'T SLOW MY THOUGHTS DOWN.
BIPOLAR - Mood Disorder Questionnaire	AT TIMES I WAS SO EASILY DISTRACTED BY THINGS AROUND ME, I HAD TROUBLE CONCENTRATING/
BIPOLAR - Mood Disorder Questionnaire	AT TIMES I HAVE FELT MUCH MORE SELF-CONFIDENT THAN USUAL.
BIPOLAR - Mood Disorder Questionnaire	AT TIMES I FELT SO GOOD OR "HYPER" THAT OTHERS THOUGHT I WAS "NOT MY NORMAL SELF
BIPOLAR - Mood Disorder Questionnaire	AT TIMES I HAD MUCH MORE ENERGY THAN USUAL.
BIPOLAR - Mood Disorder Questionnaire	AT TIMES I HAD UNUSUALLY MORE ENERGY THAN ORDINARY.
BIPOLAR - Mood Disorder Questionnaire	AT TIMES I WAS MUCH MORE ACTIVE OR "DID MORE THINGS" THAN USUAL.
BIPOLAR - Mood Disorder Questionnaire	AT TIMES I WAS MUCH MORE INTERESTED IN SEX THAN USUAL.
BIPOLAR - Mood Disorder Questionnaire	AT TIMES I DID "UNUSUAL" THINGS - FOOLISH OR RISKY OR EXCESSIVE THINGS ACCORDING TO OTHERS.
BIPOLAR - Mood Disorder Questionnaire	AT TIMES I SPENT WAY TOO MUCH MONEY WHICH GOT MY FAMILY IN TROUBLE.
BIPOLAR - Mood Disorder Questionnaire	A HEALTH PROFESSIONAL HAS TOLD ME I WAS "BIPOLAR" OR "MANIC-DEPRESSIVE.
BIPOLAR - Mood Disorder Questionnaire	I HAVE BLOOD RELATIVES DIAGNOSED AS "BIPOLAR" OR "MANIC-DEPRESSIVE"1
BIPOLAR - Mood Disorder Questionnaire	I HAVE MOOD PROBLEMS SO BAD I HAVE LOST JOBS, HURT MY FAMILY, GOT INTO LEGAL TROUBLE OR
BIPOLAR - Mood Disorder Questionnaire	AT TIMES I WAS MUCH MORE SOCIAL/ OUTGOING THAN USUAL (like TELEPHONING FRIENDS IN THE MIDDLE

DELIRIUM DSM-5 p.41	I CANNOT FOCUS ON A SUBJECT VERY WELL.
DELIRIUM DSM-5 p.41	I CAN'T EVEN WATCH TV IF THE FAMILY IS TALKING NEARBY.
DELIRIUM DSM-5 p.41	I HAVE DIFFICULTY CONCENTRATING.
DELIRIUM DSM-5 p.41	I HAVE DIFFICULTY CONCENTRATING FOR EXTENDED PERIODS OF TIME.
DELIRIUM DSM-5 p.41	I AM HYPERSENSITIVE TO LIGHT/ "GLARE".
DELIRIUM DSM-5 p.41	I AM VERY DISTRACTIBLE.
DELIRIUM DSM-5 p.41	VERY SUDDENLY I CAN GET CONFUSIONAL SPELLS.
DELIRIUM DSM-5 p.41	I HAVE DIFFICULTY CARRYING OUT EVEN SIMPLE INSTRUCTIONS.
DELIRIUM DSM-5 p.41	I HAVE HAD EPISODES OF "SLOWED THINKING" (WITHOUT ANY ALCOHOL OR DRUG USE).
DELIRIUM DSM-5 p.41	I HAVE EPISODES WHERE PEOPLE CAN'T UNDERSTAND WHAT I AM TRYING TO SAY.
DELIRIUM DSM-5 p.41	VERY SUDDENLY I HAVE SPELLS OF POOR JUDGMENT/ MEMORY PROBLEMS/ SLOWED THINKING OR
DELIRIUM DSM-5 p.41	SOMETIMES I PERCEIVE THINGS THAT ARE SO DIFFERENT FROM WHAT OTHER'S ARE SEEING.
DELIRIUM DSM-5 p.41	I CAN'T EVEN CONVERSE WITH THE FAMILY IF THE TELEVISION OR OTHERS ARE DISTRACTING ME
DELIRIUM DSM-5 p.41	I HAVE DIFFICULTY CARRYING OUT COMPLEX INSTRUCTIONS.
DELIRIUM DSM-5 p.41	VERY SUDDENLY I HAVE SPELLS OF CONFUSION ABOUT THE DATE OR "WHERE I AM".

DEPRESSION SCALE p.41		I USUALLY FEEL SO SAD MUCH OF THE TIME.
DEPRESSION SCALE p.41		I HAVE CRYING SPELLS OR FEEL LIKE IT OFTEN.
DEPRESSION SCALE p.41	X	I EAT AS MUCH AS I USED TO.
DEPRESSION SCALE p.41	X	I ENJOY LOOKING AT, TALKING TO AND BEING WITH ATTRACTIVE WOMEN/MEN.
DEPRESSION SCALE p.41		I HAVE TROUBLE SLEEPING THROUGH THE NIGHT.
DEPRESSION SCALE p.41		I NOTICE THAT I AM LOSING WEIGHT.
DEPRESSION SCALE p.41		I HAVE TROUBLE WITH CONSTIPATION.
ANZIETY - ZUNG		MY HEART BEATS FASTER THAN USUAL.
DEPRESSION SCALE p.41		I GET TIRED FOR NO REASON.
DEPRESSION SCALE p.41	X	MY MIND IS AS CLEAR AS IT USED TO BE.
DEPRESSION SCALE p.41		I FIND IT HARD TO DO THE THINGS I USED TO.
DEPRESSION SCALE p.41		I AM RESTLESS AND CAN'T KEEP STILL.
DEPRESSION SCALE p.41	X	I FEEL HOPEFUL ABOUT THE FUTURE.
DEPRESSION SCALE p.41		I AM MORE IRRITABLE THAN USUAL.
DEPRESSION SCALE p.41		I HAD A PLAN TO KILL MYSELF; STARTED TO DO IT & THEN STOPPED AT THE LAST MINUTE.
DEPRESSION SCALE p. 41		I HAVE FELT LIKE RUNNING INTO TRAFFIC.

	NEVER	SOMETIMES	OFTEN	Very Often	**COMPLAINT**
DEPRESSION SCALE p.41	X				I FIND IT EASY TO MAKE DECISIONS.
DEPRESSION SCALE p.41					I DON'T FEEL THAT I AM USEFUL OR NEEDED.
DEPRESSION SCALE p.41					MY LIFE SEEMS SO EMPTY.
DEPRESSION SCALE p.41					I FEEL THAT OTHERS WOULD BE BETTER OFF IF I WERE DEAD.
DEPRESSION SALE p.41	X				I STILL ENJOY THE THINGS I USED TO.
DEPRESSION SCALE p.41					ALMOST DAILY I THINK I WOULD BE BETTER OFF IF I WERE DEAD.
DEPRESSION SCALE p.41					I HAVE DREAMED ABOUT DEATH.
DEPRESSION SCALE p.41					I HAVE HAD IDEAS ABOUT KILLING MYSELF.
DEPRESSION SCALE p.41					I HAVE THOUGHT ABOUT DEATH AND DYING.
DEPRESSION SCALE p.41					I HAVE THOUGHT ABOUT WAYS TO KILL MYSELF.
DEPRESSION SCALE p.41					I HAVE GOTTEN SO DISCOURAGED THAT I THOUGHT ABOUT ENDING MY LIFE.
DEPRESSION SCALE p.41					I HAD A PLAN OF HOW I WOULD KILL MYSELF.
DEPRESSION SCALE p.41					I HAVE WISHED I WERE DEAD.
DEPRESSION SCALE p.41					I HAVE FELT LIKE LIFE WAS NOT WORTH LIVING.
DEPRESSION SCALE p.41					I HAVE THOUGHT ABOUT KILLING MYSELF BUT DID NOT TRY TO DO IT.
DEPRESSION SCALE p.41					I TRIED TO KILL MYSLEF.
DEPRESSION SCALE p.41					I DREAMED ABOUT KILLING MYSELF.
DEPRESSION SCALE p.41					I TALKED TO SOMEONE ABOUT KILLING MYSELF.

Drug Abuse Screening Test	I HAVE USED DRUGS OTHER THAN THOSE REQUIRED FOR MEDICAL REASONS.
Drug Abuse Screening Test	I HAVE USED MORE THAN ONE NON-PRESCRIBED DRUG AT A TIME.
Drug Abuse Screening Test	I AM UNABLE TO STOP USING DRUGS WHEN I WANT TO.
Drug Abuse Screening Test	I HAVE HAD BLACKOUTS OR FLASHBACKS AS A RESULT OF DRUG USE.
Drug Abuse Screening Test	MY LIFE PARTNER (OR PARENTS) HAVE COMPLAINED ABOUT MY INVOLVEMENT WITH DRUGS.
Drug Abuse Screening Test	I HAVE NEGLECTED MY FAMILY BECAUSE OF MY USE OF ILLEGAL DRUGS.
Drug Abuse Screening Test	I HAVE ENGAGED IN ILLEGAL ACTIVITIES IN ORDER TO OBTAIN DRUGS.
Drug Abuse Screening Test	I HAVE EXPERIENCED WITHDRAWL SYMPTOMS (FELT SICK) WHEN I STOPPED TAKING DRUGS.
Drug Abuse Screening Test	I HAVE HAD MEDICAL PROBLEMS AS A RESULT OF MY DRUG USE (e.g., MEMORY LOSS/ HEPATITIS/
Drug Abuse Screening Test	I HAVE HAD MEDICAL PROBLEMS AS A RESULT OF MY DRUG USE (e.g., MEMORY LOSS/ HEPATITIS/
Drug Abuse Screening Test	I HAVE SMOKED CIGARETTES.
Drug Abuse Screening Test	I HAVE USED ALCOHOL EXCESSIVELY.
Drug Abuse Screening Test	I HAVE DRUNK ALCOHOLIC BEVERAGES.
Drug Abuse Screening Test	I HAVE SMOKED MARIJUANA.
Drug Abuse Screening Test	I HAVE TAKEN DRUGS OTHER THAN MARIJUANA OR PRESCRIPTION DRUGS.
Epworth Sleepiness Scale	I CAN FALL ASLEEP JUST SITTING AND READING.
Epworth Sleepiness Scale	I CAN FALL ASLEEP JUST WATCHING TELEVISION.
Epworth Sleepiness Scale	I CAN FALL ASLEEP AS A PASSENGER IN A CAR FOR AN HOUR WITHOUT A BREAK.
Epworth Sleepiness Scale	I CAN FALL ASLEEP LYING DOWN TO REST IN THE AFTERNOON WHEN CIRCUMSTANCES PERMIT.
Epworth Sleepiness Scale	I CAN FALL ASLEEP JUST SITTING AND TALKING TO SOMEONE.
Epworth Sleepiness Scale	I CAN FALL ASLEEP JUST SITTING QUIETLY AFTER A LUNCH WITHOUT ALCOHOL.
Epworth Sleepiness Scale	I CAN FALL ASLEEP IN A CAR, WHILE STOPPED FOR A FEW MINUTES IN THE TRAFFIC.

DEMENTIA - Stage 2 JENICKE	I HAVE BEEN GETTING SO FORGETFUL OF APPOINTMENTS, FOR EXAMPLE WITH DOCTORS.
DEMENTIA - Stage 2 JENICKE	I HAVE BEEN GETTING SO FORGETFUL.
DEMENTIA - Stage 2 JENICKE	I HAVE BEEN GETTING SO FORGETFUL OF OTHER PEOPLE'S NAMES.
DEMENTIA - Stage 2 JENICKE	I HAVE BEEN GETTING SO FORGETFUL, I HAVE BEEN LOSING THINGS.
DEMENTIA - Stage 2 JENICKE	I HAVE BEEN GETTING SO FORGETFUL, I AM WORRIED ABOUT IT.
DEMENTIA - Stage 3 JENICKE	I HAVE BEEN GETTING SO FORGETFUL, MY CO-WORKERS HAVE NOTICED MY POOR PERFORMANCE.
DEMENTIA - Stage 3 JENICKE	I HAVE BEEN GETTING SO FORGETFUL, I HAVE DIFFICULTY FINDING THE RIGHT WORD & PEOPLES NAMES.
DEMENTIA - Stage 3 JENICKE	I HAVE BEEN GETTING SO FORGETFUL, I GET LOST WHEN TRAVELING IN UNFAMILIAR LOCATIONS.
DEMENTIA - Stage 3 JENICKE	I HAVE BEEN GETTING SO FORGETFUL, IT IS MAKING ME SO "NERVOUS".
DEMENTIA - Stage 4 JENICKE	I HAVE BEEN HAVING PROBLEMS TAKING ON NEW ASSIGNMENTS - I FEAR FAILURE.
DEMENTIA - Stage 4 JENICKE	I HAVE BEEN HAVING PROBLEMS GROWING OLD BUT I KNOW IT'S JUST NORMAL FOR MY AGE.
DEMENTIA - Stage 4 JENICKE	I HAVE BEEN HAVING PROBLEMS AT WORK AND HOME BECAUSE OF MY MEMORY.
DEMENTIA - Stage 3 JENICKE	I HAVE BEEN GETTING SO FORGETFUL PEOPLE SAY - BUT I JUST DON'T BELIEVE IT.
DEMENTIA - Stage 4 JENICKE	I HAVE BEEN HAVING PROBLEMS AT WORK AND HOME BECAUSE OF MY MEMORY.
DEMENTIA - Stage 4 JENICKE	I HAVE BEEN HAVING PROBLEMS AT WORK AND HOME BECAUSE I CAN'T CONCENTRATE ANYMORE.
DEMENTIA - Stage 4 JENICKE	I HAVE BEEN HAVING PROBLEMS AT WORK AND HOME BECAUSE I'M FORGETTING WHAT'S IN THE NEWS.
DEMENTIA - Stage 4 JENICKE	I HAVE BEEN HAVING PROBLEMS AT WORK AND HOME BECAUSE I'M FORGETTING PEOPLE'S BIRTHDAYS,
DEMENTIA - Stage 4 JENICKE	I HAVE BEEN HAVING PROBLEMS KNOWING HOW TO PAY MY BILLS NOW.
DEMENTIA - Stage 4 JENICKE	I HAVE BEEN HAVING PROBLEMS KNOWING HOW TO TRAVEL ALONE NOW - I NEED SOMEONE WITH ME.
DEMENTIA - Stage 5 JENICKE	I HAVE BEEN FORGETTING NAMES OF CLOSE FAMILY MEMBERS, TELEPHONE NUMBERS I ONCE KNEW &
DEMENTIA - Stage 5 JENICKE	I HAVE BEEN HAVING PROBLEMS TRYING TO DO THINGS WITHOUT HELP FROM OTHERS.
DEMENTIA - Stage 5 JENICKE	I HAVE BEEN GETTING CONFUSED TRYING TO BE ON TIME AND GETTING TO THE RIGHT PLACE.

DEMENTIA - Stage 5 JENICKE	I HAVE BEEN FORGETTING THE NAMES OF MY SPOUSE AND MY CHILDREN.
DEMENTIA - Stage 5 JENICKE	I HAVE BEEN FORGETTING MY OWN NAME SOMETIMES.
DEMENTIA - Stage 5 JENICKE	I HAVE BEEN FORGETTING HOW TO DRESS MYSELF CORRECTLY.
DEMENTIA - Stage 5 JENICKE	I EVEN NEED ASSISTANCE FEEDING MYSELF AND WITH MY TOILET NEEDS.
DEMENTIA - Stage 6 JENICKE	I CAN'T MAKE DECISIONS ANYMORE - IT "TAKES TOO MUCH OUT OF ME".
DEMENTIA - Stage 6 JENICKE	SOMETIMES I FORGET MY SPOUSE'S NAME.
DEMENTIA - Stage 6 JENICKE	I DON'T REMEMBER WHAT'S HAPPENING IN THE NEWS OR EVEN IN MY OWN FAMILY.
DEMENTIA - Stage 6 JENICKE	I DO REMEMBER A LITTLE BIT ABOUT MY PAST LIFE.
DEMENTIA - Stage 6 JENICKE	I DON'T PAY ATTENTION TO WHAT SEASON IT IS OR WHAT HOLIDAY IS "COMING UP".
DEMENTIA - Stage 6 JENICKE	MY SLEEP PATTERNS ARE SO DISTURBED NOW.
DEMENTIA - Stage 6 JENICKE	THEY SAY I'LL CLEAN THE HOUSE ALL DAY OR RAKE LEAVES ALL AFTERNOON - REPETITIVELY.
DEMENTIA - Stage 6 JENICKE	I'VE BEEN VERY NERVOUS AND I'VE EVEN GOTTEN VIOLENT AT TIMES.
DEMENTIA - Stage 6 JENICKE	I'VE LOST ALL MY "DRIVE" - I JUST DON'T CARE ABOUT ANYTHING ANYMORE.
DEMENTIA - Stage 7 JENICKE VERY	THEY SAY I'M SHOWING "NEUROLOGICAL SIGNS" NOW.
DEMENTIA - Stage 6 JENCKE	I'M NOT SURE THE PERSON LIVING WITH ME IS REALLY MY SPOUSE - IT DOESN'T SEEM POSSIBLE.
DEMENTIA - Stage 7 JENICKE VERY	I'VE LOST THE ABILITY TO COMMUNICATE NOW.
DEMENTIA - Stage 7 JENICKE VERY	I HAVE TO HAVE HELP FEEDING MYSELF AND GOING TO THE TOILET.
DEMENTIA - Stage 7 JENICKE VERY	I HAVE MUCH TROUBLE WALKING PROPERLY NOW.
DEMENTIA - Stage 6 JENICKE	PEOPLE SAY MY "PERSONALITY" HAS CHANGED SO MUCH.

DEMENTIA - Stage 7 JENICKE VERY	THEY SAY I'M CRAZY" BECAUSE I SMELL "STRANGE SMELLS" SOMETIMES.
DEMENTIA - Stage 7 JENICKE VERY	THEY SAY I'M CRAZY" BECAUSE I "SEE THINGS" - THAT OTHERS DON'T SEE.
DEMENTIA - Stage 7 JENICKE VERY	I'VE LOST THE ABILITY TO "HOLD MY URINE" NOW.
DEMENTIA - Stage 7 JENICKE VERY	THEY SAY I'M CRAZY" BECAUSE I "HEAR VOICES" SOMETIMES.
DEMENTIA - Stage 7 JENICKE VERY	THEY SAY I'M CRAZY" BECAUSE I "SEE THINGS" - (LIGHTS & COLORS) THAT OTHERS DON'T SEE
DEMENTIA - Stage 7 JENICKE VERY	THEY SAY I'M CRAZY" BECAUSE I SUSPECT CONSPIRACIES THAT OTHERS DON'T UNDERSTAND
DEMENTIA - Stage 7 JENICKE VERY	THEY SAY I'M CRAZY" BECAUSE I "HEAR VOICES" SOMETIMES.

FUNCTIONAL IMPAIRMENT SCALE	I HAVE DIFFICULTY PRONOUNCING WORDS CLEARLY SO OTHERS CAN UNDERSTAND ME.
FUNCTIONAL IMPAIRMENT SCALE	I CAN GET OUT OF BED ON TIME.
FUNCTIONAL IMPAIRMENT SCALE	I CAN WALK FAR FROM HOME
FUNCTIONAL IMPAIRMENT SCALE	I AM ABLE TO VISIT A FRIEND WHEN I WANT TO.
FUNCTIONAL IMPAIRMENT SCALE	I CAN SHOP FOR MY FOOD.
FUNCTIONAL IMPAIRMENT SCALE	I CAN SHOP IN THE STORES FOR MY CLOTHES.
FUNCTIONAL IMPAIRMENT SCALE	I CAN CORRECTLY PAY THE BILLS.
FUNCTIONAL IMPAIRMENT SCALE	I CAN MAKE CORRECT CHANGE.
FUNCTIONAL IMPAIRMENT SCALE	I CAN BALANCE A CHECKBOOK.
FUNCTIONAL IMPAIRMENT SCALE	I CAN RIDE A BICYCLE.
FUNCTIONAL IMPAIRMENT SCALE	I CAN DRIVE A CAR.
FUNCTIONAL IMPAIRMENT SCALE	I CAN TAKE THE BUS BY MYSELF.
FUNCTIONAL IMPAIRMENT SCALE	I HAVE A CURRENT DRIVER'S LICENSE.
FUNCTIONAL IMPAIRMENT SCALE	I AM ABLE TO STAY OVERNIGHT AT A FRIEND'S HOUSE.
FUNCTIONAL IMPAIRMENT SCALE	I CAN COOK A WHOLE MEAL BY MYSELF.
FUNCTIONAL IMPAIRMENT SCALE	I CAN CLEAN MY ROOMS.
FUNCTIONAL IMPAIRMENT SCALE	I CAN DO THE DISHES.
FUNCTIONAL IMPAIRMENT SCALE	I CAN CLEAN THE WHOLE HOUSE.
FUNCTIONAL IMPAIRMENT SCALE	I CAN CLEAN THE YARD.
FUNCTIONAL IMPAIRMENT SCALE	I CAN WORK AT ASSISTED LIVING.
FUNCTIONAL IMPAIRMENT SCALE	I CAN WORK AT A REGULAR JOB.
FUNCTIONAL IMPAIRMENT SCALE	I CAN READ FROM A BOOK.

FUNCTIONAL IMPAIRMENT SCALE	I CAN READ FROM A BOOK AND REMEMBER MUCH.
FUNCTIONAL IMPAIRMENT SCALE	I CAN WATCH TV AND REMEMBER MUCH.
FUNCTIONAL IMPAIRMENT SCALE	I CAN DISCUSS CURRENT EVENTS WITH FRIENDS.
FUNCTIONAL IMPAIRMENT SCALE	I CAN SOLVE SOME DIFFICULT PROBLEMS.
FUNCTIONAL IMPAIRMENT SCALE	I CAN INITIATE A CONVERSATION WITH FRIENDS.
FUNCTIONAL IMPAIRMENT SCALE	I CAN INITIATE A CONVERSATION WITH STRANGERS.
FUNCTIONAL IMPAIRMENT SCALE	I CAN GUESS CORRECTLY WHAT YOU ARE "FEELING" INSIDE..
FUNCTIONAL IMPAIRMENT SCALE	I CAN CARE ABOUT OTHERS.
FUNCTIONAL IMPAIRMENT SCALE	I CAN VOTE AT ELECTION TIME.
FUNCTIONAL IMPAIRMENT SCALE	I CAN WORK WITH TOOLS.
FUNCTIONAL IMPAIRMENT SCALE	I CAN WORK WITH COMPUTERS.
FUNCTIONAL IMPAIRMENT SCALE	I CAN USE CORRECT ENGLISH.
FUNCTIONAL IMPAIRMENT SCALE	I HAVE DIFFICULTY FOLLOWING THROUGH AND "FINISHING" PROJECTS.
FUNCTIONAL IMPAIRMENT SCALE	I CAN USE CORRECT ENGLISH.
FUNCTIONAL IMPAIRMENT SCALE	I HAVE DIFFICULTY PLANNING AND ORGANIZING THINGS.
FUNCTIONAL IMPAIRMENT SCALE	I HAVE DIFFICULTY THINKING CLEARLY AND EFFICIENTLY.
FUNCTIONAL IMPAIRMENT SCALE	I HAVE DIFFICULTY READING AND WRITING.
REPRESSION (F) NEVER	SOMETIMES I DO TELL LITTLE LIES.
REPRESSION (F) NEVER	I PREFER TO WIN RATHER THAN LOSE WHEN I PLAY GAMES.
REPRESSION (T) VERY OFTEN	I LIKE EVERYONE I KNOW.
REPRESSION (F) NEVER	SOMETIMES I GET ANGRY.

Ch. 2: Health History/ R.O.S.

PLACE	AN "X" MARK IF YOU	HAVE	THIS	PROBLEM	"VERY OFTEN"	"SOMETIMES"	"NEVER"
Feeling sad,	depressed or hopeless	____	____	_____			
Getting mad/	irritated, & explosive	____	__	_____			
So "stressed	out" I have "ringing in	the	ears"	_____			
So angry that	I could kill someone __	____	_ ___	_____			
So sad I can	kill myself _____	____	____	_____			
People have	teased & bullied me __	____	____	_____			
Some people	sexually molested me	____	____	_____			
I have teased	& bullied others _____	____	____	_____			
People have	lied to me so much	____	____	_____			
I make sure I	never tell a lie _____	____	____	_____			
People will	abuse you if they can	____	____	_____			
I feel like	"nobody really cares"	____	____	_____			
I get dizzy,	headaches, nervous, or	short	of	breath _____			
I get very bad	stomachaches _____	____	____	_____			
I can not pay	attention like I used to	____	____	_____			
I get more	"jumpy"/ startled now	____	____	_____			
I have been	having nightmares ___	____	____	_____			
People say I	"daydream" a lot _____	____	____	_____			
I feel strange	"tingling" in my body	____	____	_____			
I abuse	alcohol/drugs/MJ, etc	____	____	_____			
I have been	having sex with others	____	____	_____			
I am failing at	school _____	____	____	_____			
I have chest	pains_____	____	____	_____			
I have had	head injuries _____	____	____	_____			
I see ghosts	or "strange shadows"	____	____	_____			
I hear things	even when alone	____	____	_____			
I prefer to be	alone in my room	____	____	_____			
I don't have	any friends.	____	____	_____			

PROBLEM NOTED	THE PROBLEM STARTED-			NOW THE PROBLEM IS-			
	AT BIRTH	YEARS AGO	IN PAST FEW MONTHS	NO LONGER PRESENT	GETTING BETTER	STAYING THE SAME	GETTING WORSE
Ears: abnormally shaped							
Ears: much wax in canals							
Ear infections often: with fever							
Ear canal infections: without fever							
Ear: fluid or "glue ear"							
Earaches: frequent							
Hearing difficulty or deafness							
Ringing in ears							
Ear drainage of pus							
Eyes: abnormal looking							
Eyes: small eyeballs							
Eyes: extremely large or protruding							
Pupils very large							
Pupils very small							
Pupils abnormal							
Eyes: crossed: turning in							
Eyes turning out abnormally							
Eyes: excessive watering or tears							
Eyes: pus or infection							
Eyes: very red							
Eyes: very itchy							
Eyes: purple ring around iris (center)							
Eyes: pain or burning							
Trouble seeing far away things							
Trouble seeing things up close							
Blind spots with some vision							
Blindness							
Seeing double=blurred vision							
Wears glasses							
Has astigmatism							
Sees flashing lights or zig-zags							
Color-blind							
Night-vision problems							
Sensitive to the light							
Seeing visual patterns or pictures (daytime)							
Nightmares or night terrors							
Cataracts							

PROBLEM NOTED	THE PROBLEM STARTED-			NOW THE PROBLEM IS-			
	AT BIRTH	YEARS AGO	IN PAST FEW MONTHS	NO LONGER PRESENT	GETTING BETTER	STAYING THE SAME	GETTING WORSE
Excessively fearful or worried							
Compulsive, perfectionistic							
Guilt-ridden							
Hallucinating (hearing "voices")							
Head-banging							
Cries much							
Hoarse voice; whisper voice							
Gaining weight too fast							
Losing weight; not gaining							
Growing tall too fast							
Not growing fast enough							
Hungry all the time							
Never seems to be hungry							
Eats too much							
Eats too little							
Drinks too much							
Drinks too little							
Chews on paint, plaster or dirt							
Has fever							
Frequent, unexplained fevers							
Has chills or shivering spells							
Sweats very much							
Is intolerant of heat							
Is intolerant of cold							
Seems sluggish or slow							
Has a strange body odor							
Anemic: low blood count							
Gets infections very easily							
Low intelligence							
Too much blood							
Enlarged glands (neck, belly, etc.)							
Bleeds too easily or too long							
Weak: fatigue much of time							
Head: abnormally small							
Head: abnormally large							
Head: abnormally shaped							
Face: strange looking							

PROBLEM NOTED	THE PROBLEM STARTED-			NOW THE PROBLEM IS-			
	AT BIRTH	YEARS AGO	IN PAST FEW MONTHS	NO LONGER PRESENT	GETTING BETTER	STAYING THE SAME	GETTING WORSE
Nose: abnormally shaped							
Nose: excessive mucous secretions							
Nose: foul-smelling discharge							
Nose: watery discharge							
Nosebleeds, frequent							
Nose: polyps or tumors inside							
Nose itches frequently							
Nose: pain in or around							
Nose: infections							
Noisy breathing or snoring							
Sense of smell lost							
Smelling strange smells which aren't there							
Sore mouth or tongue							
Sore throat: "strep throat" frequently							
Difficulty swallowing							
Tonsils too large							
Tonsils, infected							
Teeth: abnormal							
Teeth: cavities							
Tongue: very large							
Tongue: very red or "beefy"							
Drooling saliva from mouth							
Strange odor from mouth							
Bad taste in mouth							
Loss of sense of taste							
Throat or mouth injury							
Jaw stiffness: difficulty opening							
Neck: lumps at side or back							
Neck: lump in center							
Neck pain or stiffness on moving							
Neck injury							
Difficulty breathing							
Breathes too fast							
Breathes too slowly							
Wheezes or noisy breathing							
Croup or noisy inspiration							
High blood pressure							
Low blood pressure							
Night sweats							

PROBLEM NOTED	THE PROBLEM STARTED-			NOW THE PROBLEM IS-			
	AT BIRTH	YEARS AGO	IN PAST FEW MONTHS	NO LONGER PRESENT	GETTING BETTER	STAYING THE SAME	GETTING WORSE
Overactive, restless, fidgety							
Explosive, irritable, unpredictable							
Aggressive, hostile, destructive							
Short Attention span, distractible							
Can't get to sleep							
Sleeps too much							
Seizures: jerking or stiffening							
Staring spells							
Dreamy states: automatic movements							
Falling or head-nodding spells							
Blackouts							
Dizziness or head spinning around							
Clumsiness, uncoordinated							
Muscle weakness							
Muscles, paralyzed							
Muscles, wasting away							
Muscle twitches; abnormal movements							
Tremor of hands or fingers							
Slurred speech							
Difficulty speaking							
Immature language							
Difficulty thinking							
Confusion							
Unconsciousness spells							
Poor memory; forgetting							
Poor handwriting							
Poor reading or spelling							
Numbness or tingling sensations							
Loss of sensation							
Pain, severe							
Withdrawn							
Depressed							
Excessively silly or inappropriate							
Stubborn, defiant							

PROBLEM NOTED	THE PROBLEM STARTED-			NOW THE PROBLEM IS-			
	AT BIRTH	YEARS AGO	IN PAST FEW MONTHS	NO LONGER PRESENT	GETTING BETTER	STAYING THE SAME	GETTING WORSE
Pain when breathing							
Stops breathing for long periods of time							
Cough, dry							
Coughs up clear sputum							
Coughs up yellow or green sputum							
Coughs up blood							
Coughs after eating or drinking							
Chest was injured							
Pneumonia							
Asthma							
Bronchitis							
Emphysema							
Other chest disease							
Gets short of breath at rest							
Gets short of breath on exertion							
Awakens from sleep, short of breath							
Chest pain							
Feels heart flutter or palpitations							
Heart beats too fast at times							
Heart beats too slowly at times							
Heart murmur							
Other heart disease							
Heart seems too large							
Likes to squat down on floor to breathe							
Gets very tired with exertion							
E.K.G. (heart test) was abnormal							
Chest X-ray was abnormal							
Breasts: painful							
Breasts: lump							
Breasts: infection							
Breasts: discharge from nipples							
Breasts: developing too fast							
Breasts: taking too long to develop							
Breasts: enlarging without reason							
Nipples: darkly pigmented							
Nipples: inverted							
Breasts: tender to touch							
Breasts: injury							

PROBLEM NOTED	THE PROBLEM STARTED-			NOW THE PROBLEM IS-			
	AT BIRTH	YEARS AGO	IN PAST FEW MONTHS	NO LONGER PRESENT	GETTING BETTER	STAYING THE SAME	GETTING WORSE
Painful urination							
Urinating more frequently than normal							
Wets his clothes: daytime							
Wets the bed at night							
Difficulty with urination							
Urinates too little or too seldom							
Blood in urine							
Urine: very dark-colored							
Urine: very light, like water							
Infections of kidney or bladder							
Injury to kidneys or bladder							
Kidney or bladder stones or gravel							
Tumors of kidney or bladder							
Pubic hair present too early							
BOYS: infection of penis							
BOYS: penis abnormal							
BOYS: penis injury							
BOYS: penis: too large for age							
BOYS: penis: too small for age							
BOYS: testes, infection							
BOYS: testes; abnormal							
BOYS: testes; injury							
BOYS: testes; too large for age							
BOYS: testes; too small for age							
BOYS: testes; not present; one or both sides							
GIRLS: clitoris; too large for age							
GIRLS: vagina; too developed for age							
GIRLS: menstrual bleeding too early for age							
GIRLS: menstrual bleeding too late for age							
GIRLS: menstrual bleeding; too much							
GIRLS: menstrual bleeding; too often							
GIRLS: menstrual bleeding; too seldom							
GIRLS: vaginal discharge							
GIRLS: pregnant							
GIRLS: can't get pregnant							
Masturbates in public							
Has sexually assaulted others							
Has been raped							
Injury to sexual organs							
Painful menstruation							

PROBLEM NOTED	THE PROBLEM STARTED-			NOW THE PROBLEM IS-			
	AT BIRTH	YEARS AGO	IN PAST FEW MONTHS	NO LONGER PRESENT	GETTING BETTER	STAYING THE SAME	GETTING WORSE
Stomach pain							
Nausea (feeling sick in stomach)							
Indigestion							
Vomiting							
Vomiting blood							
Gas in stomach or intestines							
Stomach bloated or enlarged							
Diarrhea (loose, frequent stools)							
Diarrhea with pus in bowel movement							
Diarrhea with fatty, floating feces							
Constipation: hard, infrequent feces							
Diarrhea with blood							
Formed bowel movement with blood							
Colic or cramps							
Stomach tenderness to touch							
Stomach tumor or lump							
Stomach, infection							
Stomach, injury							
Bowel movement: painful							
Feces: black or clay-colored							
Feces: too large or bulky							
Feces: can't be passed							
Feces: can't be controlled: soiling							
Feces: change of size: pencil-thin							
Rectum: itching							
Rectum: hemmorhoids							
Rectum: infection or worms							
Rectum: injury							
Rectum: tumors or warts							
Has ulcers							
Has colitis							
Has gallbladder disease							
Other disease of stomach area							

THE PATIENT HAS SHOWN THE FOLLOWING PROBLEMS:	THE PROBLEM STARTED			NOW THE PROBLEM IS -			
	AT BIRTH	YEARS AGO	IN PAST FEW MONTHS	NO LONGER PRESENT	GETTING BETTER	STAYING THE SAME	GETTING WORSE
Uncontrollable anger much of the time							
Elated, wild excitement, "on a high", unusually happy							
Volatile moods: changing quickly from happy to angry or sad							
Facial expression inappropriate/detached from conversation							
Anxious or worried - about everything or almost all the time							
Depressed, sad or despondent							
Anxious or worried about a specific problem							
Fearful about everything or almost all the time							
Fearful of a specific thing or event							
Distrustful & suspicious (without cause) or hypersensitive							
Hostile, negativistic or bitter							
Homocidal -wanting to kill, maim or harm others							
Suicidal - wanting to kill, maim or harm self							
Guilt-ridden, overly conscientious, excessively scrupulous							
Feeling isolated, rejected or hurt by others							
Believes his thoughts escape aloud from his head							
Believes his thoughts, impulses or acts come from another person							
Believes he is controlled by an outside force							
Has a private interpretation of reality - not shared by others							
Has fixed beliefs in conflict with reality							
Reaches conclusions in a logically unacceptable basis							
Tolerates conflicting impossibilities							
Personalizes events into a web of conspiracy against him							
Shows disorganized, shallow and silly thinking							
Is vain, self-centered or narcissistic							
Is selfish & very inconsiderate of the feelings of others							
Is disloyal, calloused & irresponsible							
Is unreliable, weak or dependent & clinging on others							
Is inflexible, rigid or has difficulty tolerating new ideas							
Is jealous & very envious: backbites & belittles others much							
Is excessively preoccupied with his own self-importance							
Ascribes evil motives to other people's actions							
Is preoccupied with sex, homosexuality or perversions							
Is preoccupied with other "obsessions" - thinks of little else							
Has lost all interest in sex: very low sex drive							
Denies his current problems have psychiatric significance							
Is unaware he has a mental problem or needs psychiatric help							
Blames others for his acts: won't take responsibility for them							

THE PATIENT HAS SHOWN THE FOLLOWING PROBLEMS:	THE PROBLEM STARTED			NOW THE PROBLEM IS -			
	AT BIRTH	YEARS AGO	IN PAST FEW MONTHS	NO LONGER PRESENT	GETTING BETTER	STAYING THE SAME	GETTING WORSE
Has visual hallucinations: sees things that aren't there							
Hears imaginary voices talking to him							
Erroneously believes he has cancer or other diseases							
Truly believes he is worthless							
Erroneously believes he has special, magical powers							
Erroneously believes famous people know him & talk to him							
Believes he has been chosen by God as a Messiah or leader							
Erroneously believes others are "after him" or persecuting him							
Is destructive & aggressive: assaults others							
Is loud, flighty, erratic or unpredictable							
His conversation jumps from one topic to another, unrelated topic							
Is overtalkative & incoherent							
Is mute: often silent or speechless							
Seems perplexed: shows bizarre postures or sits motionless							
Does bizarre, infantile or very inappropriate things							
Seems in a dream-like trance - staring for long periods							
Has shown multiple personalities - "Dr. Jekyl - Mr. Hyde"							
Walks in his sleep - is unaware of who he/she is							
Is theatrical, overly dramatic or attention-seeking							
Is seductive - trying to sexually attract indiscriminately							
Sexually exposes self - or wanders naked							
Is impotent or frigid (unable to have an erection)							
Is promiscuous/sexually indiscriminate: sleeps with anyone							
Sexually molests others - rape or child molestation							
Has bizarre compulsions: e.g., washing hands over & over again							
Very impulsive - doesn't think before he acts							
Breaks the law - in conflicts with society: always in trouble							
Lacks loyalty to persons, groups or social values							
Can't learn from past experiences							
Is remorseless: feels no guilt for his crimes							
Can't hold a job: is shiftless							
Lacks stamina or perseverance							
Obstructive, procrastinating or deliberately inefficient							
Has great difficulty showing aggression or anger							
Avoids close or competitive relationships							
Difficulty sleeping: awakens in middle of the night							
Abuses drugs							
Overuses alcohol							
Difficulty getting along with people							
Frequent money troubles, bankruptcy or bouncing checks							
Has had frequent lawsuits							
Gets wild business schemes - has far-fetched ideas							

DIZZINESS QUESTIONNAIRE for _____
Name of Patient
please make a checkmark (X) in the appropriate boxes to describe the onset & duration of the attacks:

description of the problem	The Problem Started			Now The Problem Is			
	at birth	Years Ago	In Past Few Months	gone	getting better	staying the same	getting worse
FEEL DIZZY							
FEEL LIGHT-HEADED							
FEEL LIKE FAINTING							
FEEL EVERYTHING IS BLACKING OUT							
FEEL FALLING TO THE GROUND							
ACTUALLY FALL TO THE GROUND							
BECOME UNCONSCIOUS ("BLACK OUT")							
FEEL LIKE THE ROOM IS SPINNING AROUND							
FEEL LIKE THE FLOOR IS MOVING UNDER FOOT							
FEEL VERY FRIGHTENED							
FEEL A PANIC-LIKE FEELING							
FEEL PALPITATIONS ("FLUTTERING IN CHEST")							
FEEL LIKE MY HEART IS BEATING TOO FAST							
GET VERY SWEATY - FLUSHED IN THE FACE							
TURN VERY PALE							
FEEL LIKE VOMITING							
FEEL TINGLING/NUMBNESS AROUND LIPS							
FEEL TINGLING/NUMBNESS OF HANDS/FEET							
FEEL CONFUSED							
GET A HEADACHE							
GET PARALYZED							
LOSE ABILITY TO SPEAK CLEARLY							
LOSE ABILITY TO HEAR CLEARLY							
SEE "DOUBLE" OR BLURRY THINGS							
LOSE SOME VISUAL ABILITY							
GET CHEST PAINS							
GET SHORT OF BREATH/ "SHORT-WINDED"							
GET VERY WEAK							
GET RINGING IN THE EARS							
GET A "FULLNESS FEELING" IN THE EAR							
FEEL NAUSEA OR "SICK IN THE STOMACH"							
FEEL "NERVOUSNESS" OR AGITATED							
FEEL VERY HUNGRY							
GET VOMITING SPELLS							
FEEL VERY SLEEPY WITH SPELLS							
GET SHAKING HANDS OR FINGERS							
GET STARING SPELLS							
GET DIZZY SPELLS IN BETWEEN FALLING SPELLS							
GET CONVULSIONS OR EPILEPTIC FITS							

HEALTH HISTORY   PATIENT OR PARENT QUESTIONNAIRE   PAGE 9.

INSTRUCTIONS: Place a check (X) in the appropriate box stating which relatives of the patient had the following problems:

PATIENT'S RELATIVE	HEALTH PROBLEMS WHICH THE PATIENT'S RELATIVE HAD:								
	READING/ SPELLING PROBLEM	CONVULSIONS OR EPILEPSY	INHERITED OR FAMILY DISEASES	NERVOUS BREAKDOWN	MENTAL RETARD- ATION	ASTHMA OR ALLERGY	DIABETES	TUBERCU- LOSIS	BLEEDING TENDENCY
Mother									
Father									
Brothers									
Sisters									
Aunts									
Uncles									
Cousins									
Mother's mother									
Mother's father									
Father's mother									
Father's father									

INSTRUCTIONS: Circle any of the following diseases which the patient has had: RHEUMATIC FEVER   SAINT VITUS DANCE

"RED MEASLES"   MUMPS   CHICKENPOX   ROSEOLA   WHOOPING COUGH   GERMAN (THREE DAY) MEASLES   HEPATITIS   SCARLET FEVER

HAS THE PATIENT EVER BEEN IN THE HOSPITAL?_____ FOR WHAT?_____

HAS THE PATIENT EVER HAD SURGERY?_____ FOR WHAT?_____

INSTRUCTIONS: Give the year when the patient received his vaccination or immunization for the following diseases:

SMALLPOX VACCINATION_____ DPT_____ MEASLES_____ POLIO_____

Did patient receive all three DPT shots (Diphtheria, Lockjaw, Whooping Cough)?_____

                                                                  Give date of last booster:_____
#1_____ #2_____ #3_____

Has the patient had all three doses of polio vaccine by mouth?_____

SKIN TEST FOR TUBERCULOSIS? GIVE DATE_____ WAS IT ABNORMAL IN ANY WAY?_____

DOES THE PATIENT TAKE VITAMINS?_____ WHAT KIND?_____ HOW MUCH?_____

CLIENT: _____ DATE: _____

"X" if true	YEAR	FALLING / FAINTING / DIZZY SPELL
☐		FALLING EPISODE; **NOT** ASSOCIATED WITH "**PASSING OUT**"
☐		FALLING **ONLY WHEN TRIPPING** ON SOMETHING (CARPET OR CURB)
☐		FALLING **ONLY WHEN INTOXICATED.**
☐		FALLING ASSOCIATED WITH BRIEF **UNSTEADY WALK** "Like a drunk".
☐		FALLING ASSOCIATED WITH **DIZZINESS/ "ROOM SPINNING AROUND"**
☐		FALLING AFTER **STRONG EMOTION/ LAUGHTER**
☐		FALLING SUDDENLY WITH **PARALYSIS / DIFFICULTY GETTING UP**
☐		FALLING SPELLS ASSOCIATED WITH **APNEA / BAD SNORING PROBLEM**
☐		FALLING WITH PRECEDING "**LIGHT-HEADEDNESS**"/ NAUSEA/ TREMOR
☐		FALLING PRECEDED BY RAPID **EXHAUSTION AFTER EXERCISE**
☐		FALLING **AFTER REST** (FOLLOWING EXERCISE/BIG MEAL)
☐		FALLING AFTER **EXPOSURE TO COLD**
☐		FALLING WHEN **MOVING SUDDENLY**
☐		FALLING ASSOCIATED WITH **INABILITY TO GRIP OR CHEW**
☐		FALLING IF **NECK IS SUDDENLY TURNED** OR MASSAGED
☐		
☐		FALLING **ASSOCIATED WITH "PASSING OUT"/ SEIZURES/URINATING**
☐		"PASSING OUT" **WITH FACE TURNING BLUE then FLUSHED**
☐		FALLING ASSOCIATED WITH **LOSS OF CONSCIOUSNESS**
☐		FALLING WITH **LOSS OF SPEECH/ HAND MOVEMENTS**
☐		FALLING & **UNSTEADY WALK "LIKE A DRUNK" IS ALWAYS PRESENT**
☐		FALLING ASSOCIATED WITH "**BAD HEADACHE**" AFTERWARDS
☐		FALLING WHEN HAVING **RECURRENT SEIZURES**
☐		FALLING ONLY BECAUSE **MEDICATIONS** LOWER BLOOD PRESSURE
☐		FALLING ASSOCIATED WITH **CONFUSION SPELLS/MEMORY** PROBLEMS
☐		FALLING WITH **HEART PALPITATIONS**

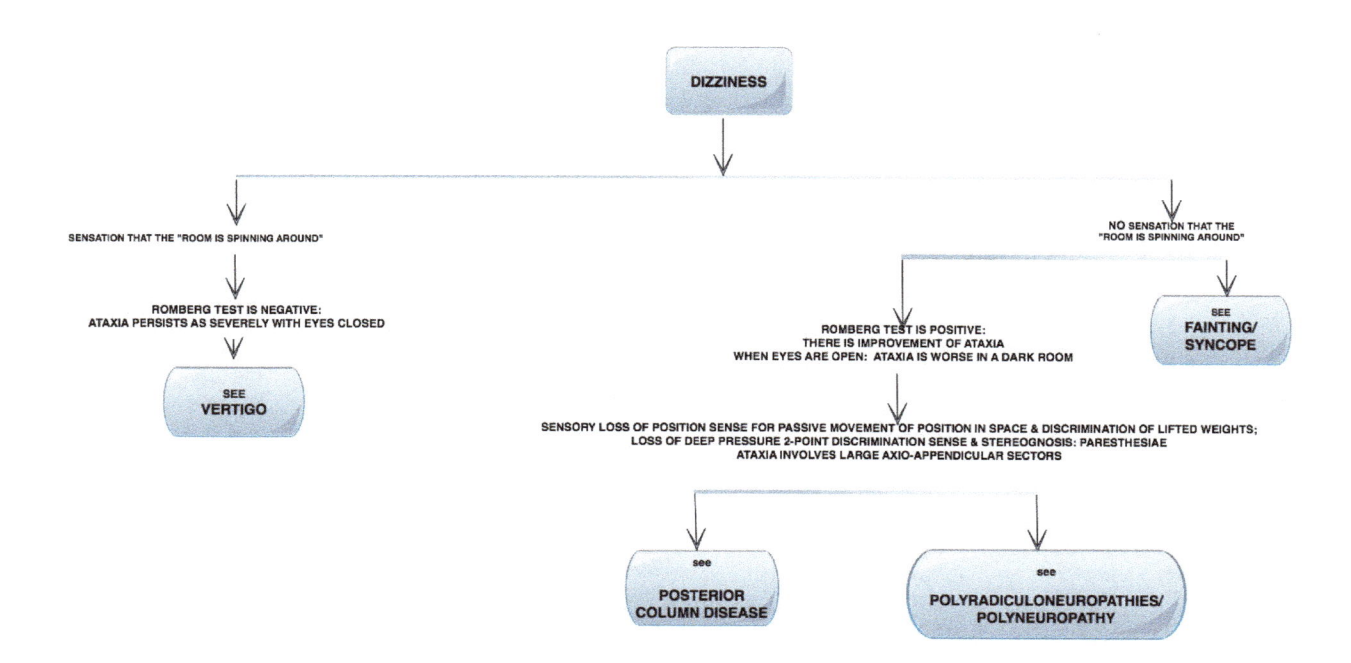

```
                        ┌─────────────┐
                        │  DIZZINESS  │
                        └──────┬──────┘
                               │
         ┌─────────────────────┼─────────────────────────────┐
         ▼                     ▼                             ▼
SENSATION THAT THE                                   NO SENSATION THAT THE
"ROOM IS SPINNING AROUND"                            "ROOM IS SPINNING AROUND"
         │                     │                             │
         ▼                     ▼                             ▼
ROMBERG TEST IS NEGATIVE:    ROMBERG TEST IS POSITIVE:    ┌──────────┐
ATAXIA PERSISTS AS SEVERELY  THERE IS IMPROVEMENT OF      │   SEE    │
WITH EYES CLOSED             ATAXIA WHEN EYES ARE OPEN:   │ FAINTING/│
         │                   ATAXIA IS WORSE IN A DARK ROOM│ SYNCOPE │
         ▼                            │                    └──────────┘
    ┌─────────┐                       ▼
    │   SEE   │        SENSORY LOSS OF POSITION SENSE FOR PASSIVE MOVEMENT
    │ VERTIGO │        OF POSITION IN SPACE & DISCRIMINATION OF LIFTED WEIGHTS;
    └─────────┘        LOSS OF DEEP PRESSURE 2-POINT DISCRIMINATION SENSE
                       & STEREOGNOSIS: PARESTHESIAE
                       ATAXIA INVOLVES LARGE AXIO-APPENDICULAR SECTORS
                                   │
                       ┌───────────┴────────────┐
                       ▼                        ▼
                  ┌─────────┐          ┌──────────────────────┐
                  │   see   │          │         see          │
                  │POSTERIOR│          │ POLYRADICULONEUROPATHIES/│
                  │ COLUMN  │          │    POLYNEUROPATHY    │
                  │ DISEASE │          └──────────────────────┘
                  └─────────┘
```

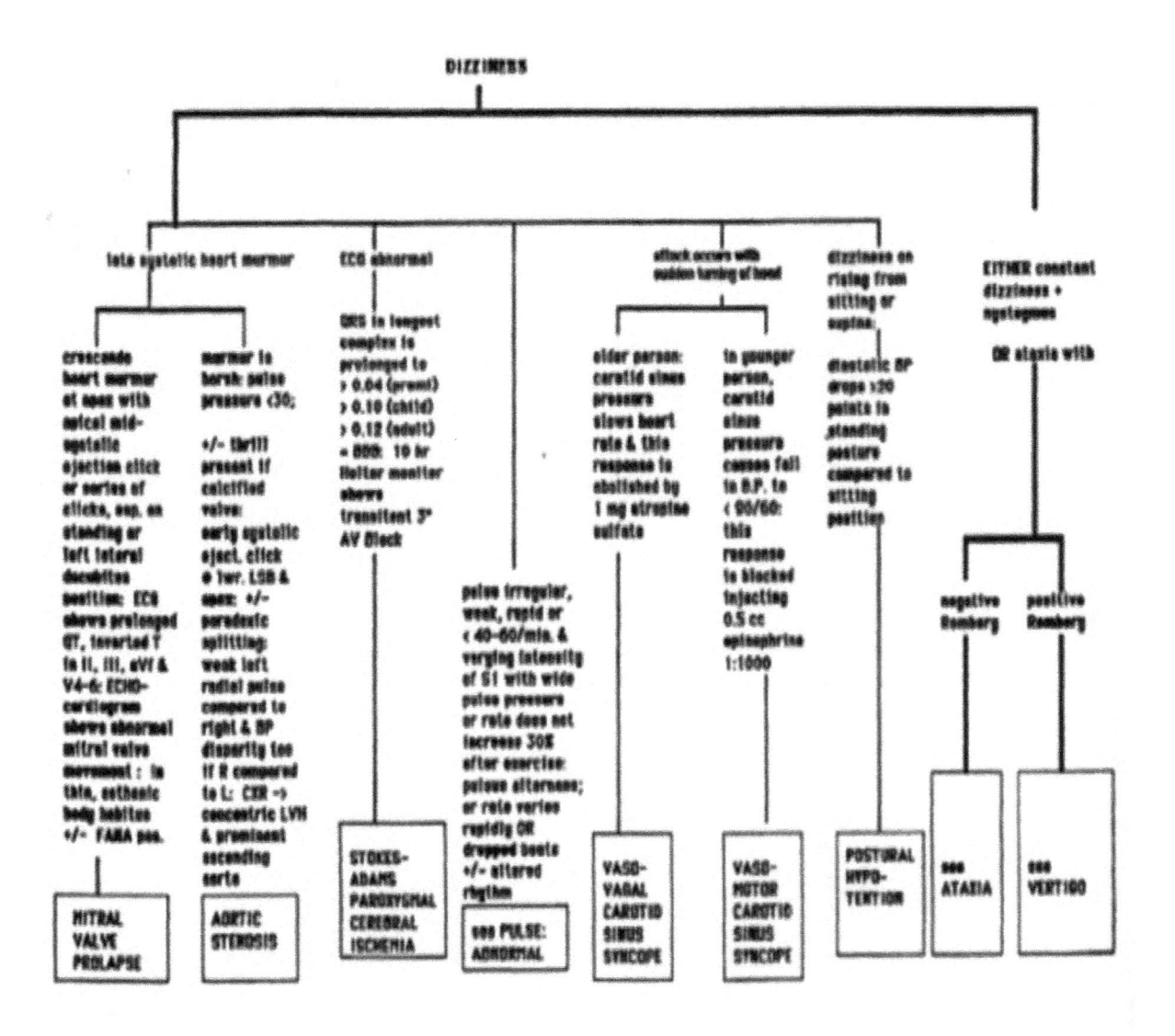

DIZZINESS

late systolic heart murmur

crescendo heart murmur at apex with apical mid-systolic ejection click or series of clicks, esp. on standing or left lateral decubitus position; ECG shows prolonged QT, inverted T in II, III, aVf & V4-6; ECHO-cardiogram shows abnormal mitral valve movement; in thin, asthenic body habitus +/- FamHx pos.

→ **MITRAL VALVE PROLAPSE**

murmur is harsh; pulse pressure <30; +/- thrill present if calcified valve; early systolic eject. click @ lwr. LSB & apex; +/- paradoxic splitting; weak left radial pulse compared to right & BP disparity too if R compared to L; CXR → concentric LVH & prominent ascending aorta

→ **AORTIC STENOSIS**

ECG abnormal

QRS in longest complex is prolonged to > 0.04 (preemie) > 0.10 (child) > 0.12 (adult) = BBB; 10 hr Holter monitor shows transient 3° AV Block

→ **STOKES-ADAMS PAROXYSMAL CEREBRAL ISCHEMIA**

pulse irregular, weak, rapid or < 40-60/min. & varying intensity of S1 with wide pulse pressure or rate does not increase 30% after exercise; pulsus alternans; or rate varies rapidly OR dropped beats +/- altered rhythm

→ **see PULSE: ABNORMAL**

attack occurs with sudden turning of head

older person: carotid sinus pressure slows heart rate & this response is abolished by 1 mg atropine sulfate

→ **VASO-VAGAL CAROTID SINUS SYNCOPE**

in younger person, carotid sinus pressure causes fall in B.P. to < 90/60; this response is blocked injecting 0.5 cc epinephrine 1:1000

→ **VASO-MOTOR CAROTID SINUS SYNCOPE**

dizziness on rising from sitting or supine;

diastolic BP drops >20 points in standing posture compared to sitting position

→ **POSTURAL HYPOTENSION**

EITHER constant dizziness + nystagmus OR ataxia with

- **negative Romberg** → see **ATAXIA**
- **positive Romberg** → see **VERTIGO**

PROBLEM CHECKLIST   (X) for _____

Please Mark an "X" if the client has shown any of these problems listed below:

_____ **SUDDEN COLLAPSE** OR LOSS OF MUSCLE STRENGTH:

    _____ **NO LOSS OF CONSCIOUSNESS**

        _____ **WITHOUT ANY WARNING**;& WITHOUT "LIGHTHEADEDNESS" OR SENSATION OF "BLACKING OUT" OR OTHER WARNING; MAY OCCUR WHETHER SITTING/ STANDING.

        _____ Also HAVING **OVERWHELMING URGE TO SLEEP IN THE DAYTIME** or "CONSTANTLY FALLING ASLEEP" IN THE DAYTIME; may have **hallucinations** WHEN FALLING ASLEEP or WHEN WAKING UP FROM SLEEP.

        _____ **WITH FEELING OF "LIGHTHEADEDNESS" & SENSATION OF "BLACKING OUT" PRIOR TO FAINTING.**

        _____ Occurs especially when suddenly getting up from a chair or "jumping out to bed"

        _____ WITH **CHEST PAINS** or "HEART PALPITATIONS" or SHORTNESS OF BREATH SPELLS.___

    _____ **WITH LOSS OF CONSCIOUSNESS**

        ____ AND STRANGE SENSATION IN TONGUE/CHEEK/GUMS/STOMACH or DROOLING/ FACIAL MOVEMENTS.

        ____ WITH VISION LOSS IN ONE EYE/ "SEEING THINGS"/ "BRIGHT/WHITE SPOTS" IN THE EYE; OR ONE-SIDED

        ____ OR **MOTOR SEIZURES ALL OVER THE BODY.**

_____ **STARING SPELLS LASTING UP TO 2 MINUTES**; not wakened by shoulder shake or hearing name

    _____ Occurs with eye-blinking/ lip-smacking or twirling one's hair or fumbling a shirt button, e.g.
        ____Several times a week OR
        ____Many times a day.

_____ **SUDDEN ONSET OF DIZZINESS/ VERTIGO; "ROOM SPINNING AROUND" SENSATION**

    _____ Associated with hearing loss & "loss of balance" sense +/- "ringing in the ears"

    _____ Occurs especially when jerking head into a certain position.

    _____ Associated with severe headache, weakness/trouble walking/speaking & confusion

_____ **FALLS FROM PROLONGED LOSS OF CONSCIOUSNESS**

_____ **FALLS FROM PROLONGED PERIODS OF MUSCLE WEAKNESS**

_____ **FALLS AFTER CHRONIC ILLNESS (SUCH AS LOW BLOOD COUNT, INFECTION, ETC)**

_____ **OTHER REASONS KNOWN TO CAUSE FALLS (E.G. BONE PROBLEMS):**

_____

Reviewed by: _____   **Date:** _____

SYNCOPE/ FAINTING

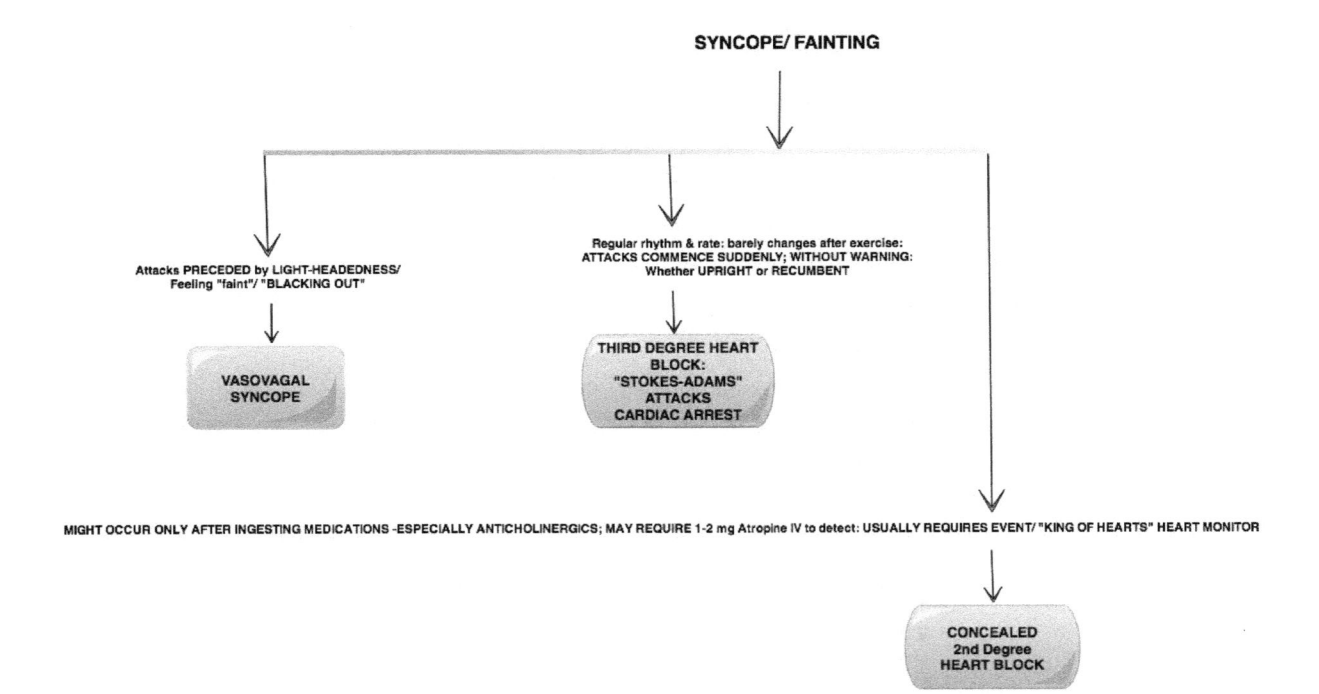

- **Attacks PRECEDED by LIGHT-HEADEDNESS/ Feeling "faint"/ "BLACKING OUT"**
  → **VASOVAGAL SYNCOPE**

- **Regular rhythm & rate: barely changes after exercise: ATTACKS COMMENCE SUDDENLY; WITHOUT WARNING: Whether UPRIGHT or RECUMBENT**
  → **THIRD DEGREE HEART BLOCK: "STOKES-ADAMS" ATTACKS CARDIAC ARREST**

- **MIGHT OCCUR ONLY AFTER INGESTING MEDICATIONS -ESPECIALLY ANTICHOLINERGICS; MAY REQUIRE 1-2 mg Atropine IV to detect: USUALLY REQUIRES EVENT/ "KING OF HEARTS" HEART MONITOR**
  → **CONCEALED 2nd Degree HEART BLOCK**

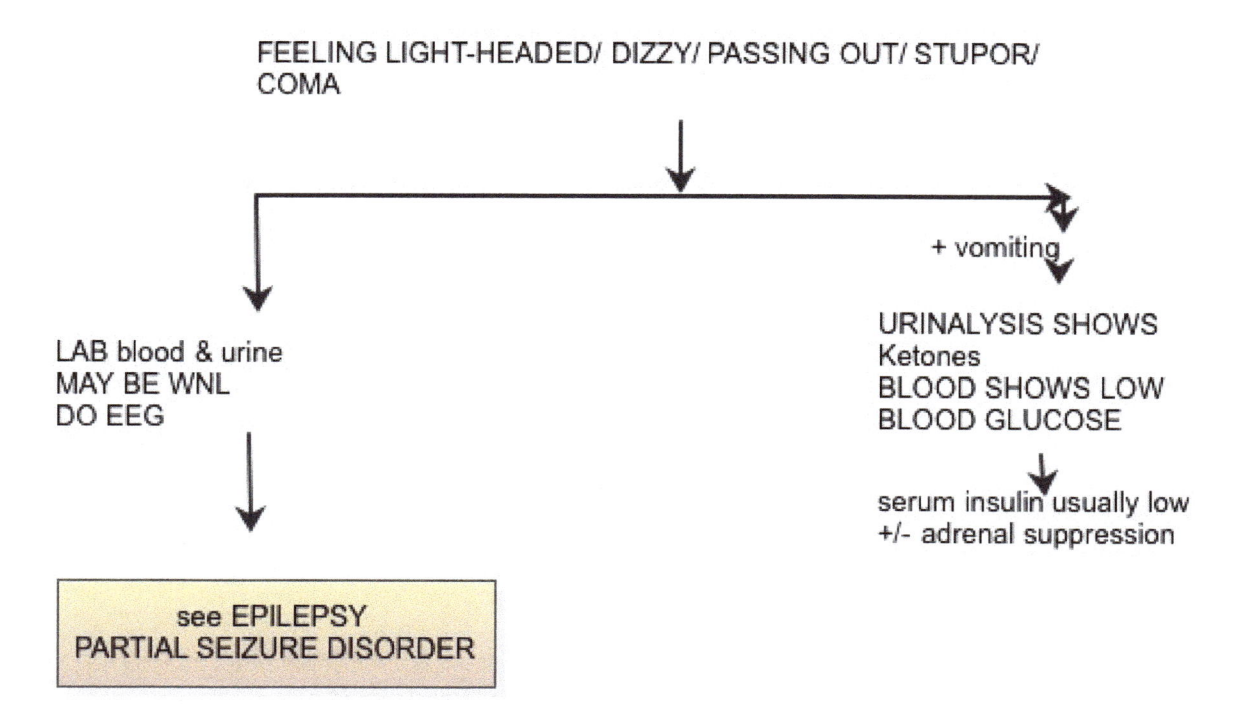

```
FEELING LIGHT-HEADED/ DIZZY/ PASSING OUT/ STUPOR/ COMA
                            │
        ┌───────────────────┴──────────────────┐
        │                                   + vomiting
        ▼                                      ▼
LAB blood & urine                    URINALYSIS SHOWS
MAY BE WNL                           Ketones
DO EEG                               BLOOD SHOWS LOW
        │                            BLOOD GLUCOSE
        │                                      │
        ▼                                      ▼
                                     serum insulin usually low
                                     +/- adrenal suppression
```

see EPILEPSY PARTIAL SEIZURE DISORDER

KETOTIC HYPOGLYCEMIA of CHILDHOOD

SEIZURE HISTORY   PARENT QUESTIONNAIRE   PAGE 1.

NAME OF PATIENT:_____ BIRTHDATE:_____

Please describe the seizure in your own words:_____
_____
_____
_____
_____
_____

List current medicines being taken for seizures: name of medicine; amount or dosage of the medicine per day and state number of days medicine was forgotten during the past month.
MEDICATION   DOSAGE   AMOUNT PER DAY   HOW MANY DAYS MEDS. FORGOTTEN PER MONTH
_____
_____
_____

GIVE THE DATE & TIME WHEN LAST SEIZURE MEDICINES WERE GIVEN & STATE AMOUNT GIVEN:_____
_____

List medicines used in the past for seizures: include the dates when these were used.
MEDICATION   DOSAGE   AMOUNT PER DAY   DATE GIVEN   RESULTS
_____
_____
_____

PLACE A CHECK (X) BEFORE ANY OF THE FOLLOWING ITEMS WHICH SEEM TO "BRING-ON" A SEIZURE:

_____ Startle (loud noises; surprise touch or movements)
_____ Fatigue (physical or emotional exhaustion)
_____ Emotional upsets
_____ Infections
_____ Fever
_____ Early sleep
_____ Waking up in the morning
_____ Flashes of light or blinking light patterns
_____ Television screen out of focus
_____ Music
_____ Some smells
_____ Sudden withdrawl from barbiturates (Phenobarbital or Seconal, e.g.) or alcohol.
_____ Not taking medication faithfully.
_____ Breath-holding
_____ Breathing too rapidly
_____ Eating or drinking certain foods or drugs
_____ Bee stings or insect bites

SEIZURE HISTORY   PAGE 2.

CHECK (X) ANY OF THE FOLLOWING WHICH OCCUR BEFORE THE SEIZURE:
_____ Visual sensations (colors, forms, shapes; things getting larger or smaller)
_____ Sounds in ears (buzzing, words, music, noises)
_____ Numbness, creeping or crawling sensations.
_____ Dizziness or twirling sensations; feeling like fainting.
_____ Queer feelings in stomach, nausea or vomiting
_____ Heart flutter, sweating or drooling
_____ Turning pale or red in the face
_____ Shivering or muscle twitches
_____ Throat spasms or being unable to breathe
_____ Knowing that a seizure is going to happen
_____ Feeling like what is happening "has happened before" - as if dreamed
_____ Dreamy feelings; lonesomeness, fearfulness or depression
_____ Weird thoughts or ideas
_____ Screaming, crying or laughing
_____ Night terrors; unable to sleep or abnormal drowsiness
_____ Hyperactivity (overly busy) or excessive irritability

CHECK (X) ANY OF THE FOLLOWING WHICH OCCUR DURING THE SEIZURE:
_____ Staring spells
_____ Eyes turn upward or blink frequently
_____ If standing, body sways back & forth
_____ Not aware of what patient is doing
_____ Lips smack & mouth shows chewing motions
_____ Hands & fingers automatically pick at clothes or objects, over & over
_____ Running or running in a circle
_____ Panic or fearfulness
_____ Anger or rage
_____ Destructive behavior or violence
_____ Head turning to one side
_____ Unconsciousness so that patient cannot be awakened (how long unconscious?_____)
_____ Urination or passing a bowel movement
_____ Tongue-biting
_____ Jerking spells of arm or leg
_____ Stiffening spells of arm or leg
_____ Jerking spells or stiffening spells of both sides of body
_____ Eyes rolling back
_____ Sudden, violent fall to floor
_____ Falling spells with immediate picking self up again
_____ Buckles over like a jack-knife
_____ Head nods; arms often raise
_____ Numbness, tingling sensations or feelings of hot & cold, etc.

CHECK (X) ANY OF THE FOLLOWING WHICH ARE PRESENT AFTER A SEIZURE
_____ Difficulty speaking clearly
_____ Difficulty thinking clearly
_____ Headaches
_____ Nausea or vomiting
_____ Difficulty moving muscles
_____ Arms are weak
_____ Legs are weak
_____ Sleepiness
_____ Bladder or bowel problems
_____ Loss of memory for the lip-smacking, chewing or automatic movements of hands
_____ Memory for the feelings of fear or rage
_____ Difficult to excite for hours after a spell
_____ Seems "washed-out" after a seizure

SEIZURE HISTORY   PARENT QUESTIONNAIRE   PAGE 3.

	STARING AND EYEBLINKING	STARING & STRANGE BEHAVIOR SPELLS	MUSCLE STIFFENING OR JERKING SPELLS	FALLING OR NODDING SPELL
AGE AT WHICH SPELLS STARTED				
AGE AT WHICH SPELLS STOPPED				
NUMBER OF SPELLS EACH DAY				
USUAL TIME OF DAY FOR SPELLS TO OCCUR: (A.M. before rising; A.M. during breakfast; afternoon; evening; during sleep)				

List any relative who had epilepsy or seizures: state whether these occurred even without fever.

RELATIVE	DIAGNOSIS	DID SEIZURES OCCUR WITHOUT FEVER?

GIVE DATE & RESULTS (NORMAL, ABNORMAL OR UNKNOWN) FOR ANY BRAIN-WAVE TEST DONE TO THE PATIENT:

DATE OF E.E.G. TEST	RESULTS	WHERE WAS TEST PERFORMED?

CIRCLE "TRUE" OR "FALSE" FOR EACH OF THE FOLLOWING STATEMENTS:

Even before the seizures, the patient seems different from his old "normal" self	FALSE	TRUE
The patient showed behavior problems even before the seizures	FALSE	TRUE
The patient has been hyperactive (overly busy) since he was an infant	FALSE	TRUE
The patient has been overactive or irritable only since the seizures started	FALSE	TRUE
The patient has been overactive only since medications were started	FALSE	TRUE
The patient has been sluggish since infancy	FALSE	TRUE
The patient got sluggish even before medications were started	FALSE	TRUE
The patient is sluggish when taking medications for seizures	FALSE	TRUE
Large muscle coordination has been getting worse these past months	FALSE	TRUE
The patient is more clumsy & falls more frequently than he used to	FALSE	TRUE
The patient complains of frequent headaches	FALSE	TRUE
The patient has been vomiting frequently in the past months or weeks	FALSE	TRUE
The patient complains of trouble with vision in the past months	FALSE	TRUE

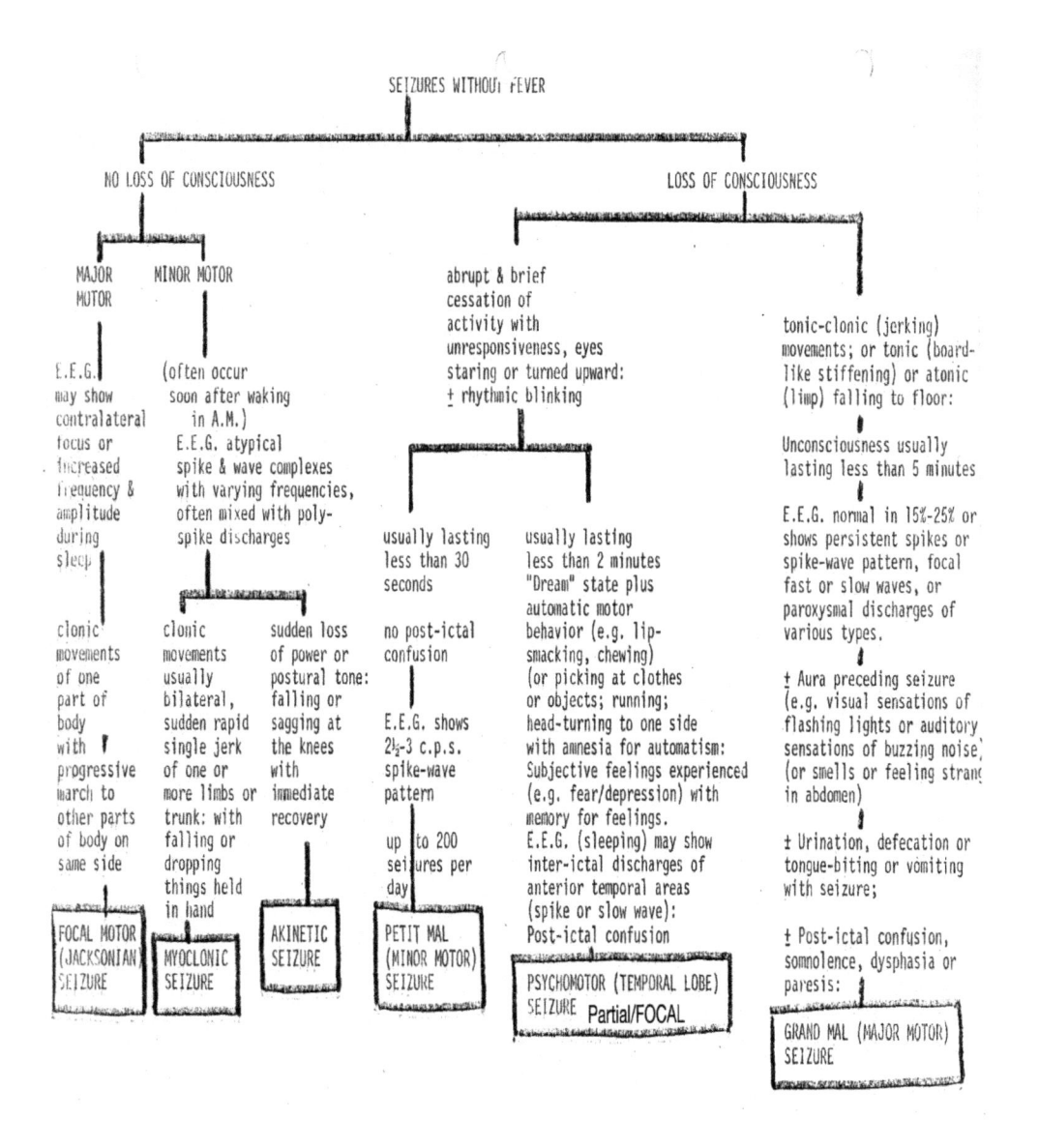

```
                                    SEIZURES WITHOUT FEVER
        ┌───────────────────────────────────────┴───────────────────────────────────────┐
   NO LOSS OF CONSCIOUSNESS                                                    LOSS OF CONSCIOUSNESS
   ┌──────────┴──────────┐                          ┌──────────────────────────────────────┴──────────┐
 MAJOR        MINOR MOTOR
 MOTOR
```

MAJOR MOTOR	MINOR MOTOR		abrupt & brief cessation of activity with unresponsiveness, eyes staring or turned upward: ± rhythmic blinking		tonic-clonic (jerking) movements; or tonic (board-like stiffening) or atonic (limp) falling to floor:
E.E.G. may show contralateral focus or increased frequency & amplitude during sleep	(often occur soon after waking in A.M.) E.E.G. atypical spike & wave complexes with varying frequencies, often mixed with poly-spike discharges				Unconsciousness usually lasting less than 5 minutes
					E.E.G. normal in 15%-25% or shows persistent spikes or spike-wave pattern, focal fast or slow waves, or paroxysmal discharges of various types.
clonic movements of one part of body with progressive march to other parts of body on same side	clonic movements usually bilateral, sudden rapid single jerk of one or more limbs or trunk: with falling or dropping things held in hand	sudden loss of power or postural tone: falling or sagging at the knees with immediate recovery	usually lasting less than 30 seconds no post-ictal confusion E.E.G. shows 2½-3 c.p.s. spike-wave pattern up to 200 seizures per day	usually lasting less than 2 minutes "Dream" state plus automatic motor behavior (e.g. lip-smacking, chewing) (or picking at clothes or objects; running; head-turning to one side with amnesia for automatism: Subjective feelings experienced (e.g. fear/depression) with memory for feelings. E.E.G. (sleeping) may show inter-ictal discharges of anterior temporal areas (spike or slow wave): Post-ictal confusion	± Aura preceding seizure (e.g. visual sensations of flashing lights or auditory sensations of buzzing noise, (or smells or feeling strange in abdomen) ± Urination, defecation or tongue-biting or vomiting with seizure; ± Post-ictal confusion, somnolence, dysphasia or paresis:
FOCAL MOTOR (JACKSONIAN) SEIZURE	**MYOCLONIC SEIZURE**	**AKINETIC SEIZURE**	**PETIT MAL (MINOR MOTOR) SEIZURE**	**PSYCHOMOTOR (TEMPORAL LOBE) SEIZURE Partial/FOCAL**	**GRAND MAL (MAJOR MOTOR) SEIZURE**

HEADACHE HISTORY   PAGE 1.

NAME OF PATIENT:_____ BIRTHDATE:_____

Please describe the headache in your own words:_____
_____
_____
_____
_____
_____

List current medicines being taken for headache: include name of medicine, when they were started, amount or dosage of the medicine and results (whether they help or not).
MEDICATION   DOSAGE   NUMBER PILLS per DAY   WHEN STARTED   RESULTS
_____
_____
_____

List medicines used in the past for headaches & state whether they helped or not.
MEDICINE   WHEN TAKEN   AMOUNT   RESULTS
_____
_____
_____

Place a check (x) before any of the following which occur 10 to 20 minutes <u>before</u> the headache:
_____ Blind spots
_____ Zig-zag patterns seen, which resemple a cavalry fort
_____ Flashing lights
_____ Numbness & tingling
_____ Visual patterns flashing before the eyes
_____ Hearing voices which aren't really there
_____ Seeing "double"
_____ Unsteadiness; loss of muscle coordination
_____ Dizziness (as if the room is spinning around)
_____ Fainting or "black-outs"
_____ An increased sense of smell
_____ An increased sense of hearing
_____ An increased sensitivity to touch

Place a check (x) before any of the following which occur <u>during</u> the headache:
_____ Sensitivity to lights
_____ Sensitivity to noise
_____ Nausea (sick feeling in stomach)
_____ Vomiting
_____ Diarrhea
_____ Cold hands & feet

HEADACHE HISTORY   PAGE 2.

Place a check (x) before any of the following which occur <u>during</u> the headache:
- _____ Tenderness over face on side of headache
- _____ Loss of muscle strength; one-sided weakness
- _____ Paralysis: inability to move some muscles on one side of body
- _____ Slurred speech
- _____ Loss of vision in one eye
- _____ Loss of hearing in one ear
- _____ Inability to move eyeballs (to "look at something" without turning head)
- _____ "Seeing double" or blurred vision
- _____ Loss of sensation of feeling on one side of body
- _____ Tingling & numbness on one side of body
- _____ Droopy eyelid
- _____ Pupils of eye getting smaller
- _____ Face flushing
- _____ Redness or pinkness in eye
- _____ Congestion in the nose
- _____ Runny nose

Place a check (x) before the statements which describe the headaches:
- _____ Headaches occur on both sides of head at the same time
- _____ Headaches occur on right side of head only
- _____ Headaches occur on left side of head only
- _____ Headaches occur sometimes on right side and at other times occur on left side
- _____ Headaches are usually in the back of the neck
- _____ Headaches are usually over the eyeball and around the eye
- _____ Headaches are usually deep inside the eye
- _____ Headaches are usually over the forehead
- _____ Headaches are usually all around the head like a hatband
- _____ Headaches are usually over the cheeks
- _____ Headaches are deep in the jaw, teeth or back of throat
- _____ Back of neck is stiff and neck hurts when it turns or bends
- _____ Headaches are a dull, nagging ache
- _____ Headaches are pulsating and throbbing
- _____ Headaches are mild
- _____ Headaches are intense
- _____ Coughing, sneezing or straining at bowel movements makes the headaches worse
- _____ Moving around and changing position makes the headaches worse
- _____ Lying quietly makes the headache worse
- _____ During sleep, the headaches waken patient
- _____ Moving around makes the pain feel less painful
- _____ Lying quietly makes the pain feel less painful
- _____ Sleep makes the headache go away
- _____ The headaches come in spasms
- _____ The headaches are constant
- _____ The headaches come in clusters, lasting for several weeks or months in time
- _____ Each headache lasts 20-30 seconds
- _____ Each headache lasts a few minutes
- _____ Each headache lasts from several minutes to 4 hours
- _____ Each headache lasts from 6 hours to 3 days

SHORTLY BEFORE THE HEADACHE DID THE PATIENT EAT ANY OF THE FOLLOWING FOODS?
- _____ Hot dogs, sausages or cured meats
- _____ Chinese food or soy sauce on food
- _____ Cold ice cream or sherbet

HEADACHE HISTORY   PAGE 3.

BEFORE THE HEADACHES STARTED, DID THE PATIENT TAKE ANY OF THE FOLLOWING:
_____ Alcoholic beverages
_____ More than 3 cups of coffee each day
_____ Amphetamines, Ritalin, Dexedrine or Benzedrine
_____ Ergot medications (for example migraine headache medicine)
_____ Tranquilizers (which ones)_____

DOES THE PATIENT TAKE ANY OF THE FOLLOWING MEDICINES:
_____ Indomethacin (for arthritis)
_____ Nitrates (for heart pains or "angina")
_____ Progesterone, birth control pills, hormones
_____ Hypertension medicine: which ones _____

WAS THE PATIENT EXPOSED TO ANY OF THE FOLLOWING SHORTLY BEFORE THE HEADACHE:
_____ Benzene
_____ Carbon monoxide (car exhaust, coal fumes in a small room without air)
_____ Carbon tetrachloride; cleaning fluid solution
_____ Insecticides; "bug-killer" sprays or solutions
_____ Batteries being burned and inhaled; or old lead paint or plaster eaten
_____ Gunpowder inhaled
_____ Any other toxic poisons: name them _____

PLACE A CHECK (X) BEFORE ANY OF THE FOLLOWING WHICH ARE ALSO PRESENT AS PROBLEMS:
_____ Recent accidental fall or injury
_____ Recent head or neck injury
_____ Infection now or recently
_____ Fever now
_____ Rash on body
_____ Sudden loss of much blood (for example, cuts or nosebleeds)
_____ Hay fever; itchy, runny nose
_____ Sinus infection or pain over nose, cheeks or behind ears
_____ Earache or ear infection
_____ Dental cavities; teeth in poor condition
_____ Turning blue; loss of oxygen or stopped breathing
_____ At very high altitude when headaches occur
_____ Anemia
_____ Convulsions or fainting
_____ Paleness and sweating
_____ Blurred vision for a long time
_____ Squinting eyes into a pinhole in order to see well
_____ Personality changes
_____ Crossed eyes: seeing "double"
_____ Vomiting
_____ Weakness
_____ Ringing in the ears
_____ High blood pressure
_____ Trouble seeing well or loss of vision
_____ Jaw pain
_____ Pain on chewing, yawning or swallowing

PLEASE MAKE ANY OTHER COMMENTS YOU WOULD LIKE: INCLUDE WHAT YOU THINK IS CAUSING THE HEADACHE:
_____
_____

HEAD INJURY EVALUATION

Name of patient:_____Unit #_____

Birthdate:_____Age:_____ Date:_____

1. When did the head injury happen? DATE_____TIME:_____
2. Did you witness the accident?_____
3. What part of the head was injured?_____
4. How did the injury occur? (Was the patient moving; for example on a bike, running, or in a car? How far was he thrown or how far did he fall? Was the object which struck him moving? How fast?, etc.)

   _____
   _____
   _____
   _____
   _____
   _____
   _____
   _____

5. Did the patient cry out or speak immediately after the injury?_____
6. Do you know if the patient was unconscious (unable to be awakened) following the injury?_____
7. If the patient was unconscious, for how long did this last? _____
8. How much blood do you think the patient lost? _____
9. SINCE THE HEAD INJURY, HAS THE PATIENT SHOWN ANY OF THE FOLLOWING COMPLAINTS:

Complaint		
Severe headache.	No	Yes
Repeated vomiting.	No	Yes
Clumsy walking.	No	Yes
Muscle weakness.	No	Yes
A fit or convulsion (jerking or "spells").	No	Yes
"Seeing double".	No	Yes
Blurred or dimmed vision	No	Yes
Drowsiness in which he can't be awakened.	No	Yes
Personality changes (for example increased irritability).	No	Yes
Speech changes (for example, slurred speech).	No	Yes
A large soft lump on the patient's head..	No	Yes
Unequal pupils (the dark area of the center of the eye).	No	Yes

ACUTE HEAD INJURY EVALUATION

Name of Patient:_____Date:_____Time:____

Caution: if nuchal rigidity is present do not disturb neck before ruling out cervical spine fracture on X-Ray.

Describe the head injury: (percussion; palpation of depressed fractures; fonatel tension and head circumference in infants; etc.):

_____
_____
_____
_____
_____

Record the following signs every 15 minutes for at least 4 exams (unless patient is deteriorating rapidly in which case call neurosurgical consult immediately):

TIME OF EXAM					
B.P.					
PULSE RATE					
PULSE QUALITY (full/thready; regular/irreg.)					
RESPIRATION RATE					
RESPIRATION QUALITY (deep/shallow; regular/irreg.)					
PUPIL SIZE mm. RIGHT SIDE____ LEFT SIDE					
PUPIL REACTIVITY R.___ TO LIGHT L.___					
FUNDI (dilated non-pulsating R.___ retinal veins? ?papilledema ?hemorrhages)					
SENSORIUM: (coma, semicoma, stupor, drowsiness or light sleep)					
OCULOMOTOR RANGE OF MOTION					
FOCAL SIGNS: SPONTANEOUS MOVEMENTS WITHDRAWAL FROM NOXIOUS STIMULI					

ACUTE HEAD INJURY - EVALUATION OF SEVERITY

DEGREE OF SEVERITY	DURATION OF LOSS OF CONSCIOUSNESS	ABNORMAL NEUROLOGICAL SIGNS	POST-TRAUMATIC PERIOD SYMPTOMS & SIGNS	DISPOSITION
MILD: Brain Concussion, ± Contusion	seconds to few minutes	no residual neurological signs	mild headache, controlled with salicylates; irritability, drowsiness; ± vomiting	Parent's checklist & telephone reports to doctor
MODERATE HEAD INJURY: some cerebral edema, contusion or laceration	several minutes to one hour	Transient abnormal findings present: (Babinski, ataxia or unsteady gait)	severe headache; irritability; drowsiness; confusion; vomiting for 12-36 hours; mild-moderate fever	X-ray skull; Hospitalize for close observation; Neurology consultation
SEVERE HEAD INJURY: Extensive Cerebral Edema	unconsciousness lasts for an hour or more; or level of consciousness progressively deteriorates after initial lucid period.	Abnormal neurological signs develop & persist for hours or forever or fluctuate	Severe recurrent or unremitting headache; mental confusion; marked variation in level of consciousness; persistent vomiting	X-ray skull; Keep close observation of vital signs; Neurosurgical consultation

SLEEP HISTORY

CLIENT:
DATE:

DETERMINE TO WHAT DEGREE .... THESE QUALITIES ARE PRESENT

	Some	Much More	Very Much
SHOWS SNORING WHEN SLEEPING	☐	☐	☐
SHOWS BREATHING DISTURBANCE AT NIGHT	☐	☐	☐
SHOWS FATIGUE DURING THE DAYTIME	☐	☐	☐
SHOWS SNORTING/GASPING OR BREATHING PAUSES DURING SLEEP	☐	☐	☐
HAS COMPELLING NEED TO SLEEP IN THE DAYTIME	☐	☐	☐
HAS BEEN GAINING EXCESSIVE WEIGHT SINCE SLEEP DISTURBANCE	☐	☐	☐
HAS FREQUENT MORNING HEADACHES	☐	☐	☐
PEOPLE HAVE SAID THAT I "STOP BREATHING" WHEN I SLEEP	☐	☐	☐
FEEL UNREFRESHED OR "TIRED" EVEN WHEN WAKING FROM SLEEP	☐	☐	☐
HAVE GOTTEN VERY FAT OVER THE PAST YEAR OR TWO	☐	☐	☐
HAVE ENLARGED TONSILS OR ADENOIDS - PEOPLE/DOCTORS NOTICED	☐	☐	☐
HAVE "HIGH BLOOD PRESSURE"/"HYPERTENSION"	☐	☐	☐
SHOWS ABNORMAL FINDINGS ON A "SLEEP STUDY THAT WAS DONE"	☐	☐	☐
GENERAL EXCESSIVE SLEEPINESS IN THE DAYTIME	☐	☐	☐
HAVE FALLEN ASLEEP AT WORK	☐	☐	☐
HAVE FALLEN ASLEEP DRIVING THE CAR OR TALKING TO FRIENDS	☐	☐	☐

Notes:

SUDDEN COLLAPSE INTO SLEEP; AROUSABLE TO NAME-CALLING;
ADEQUATE RESPONSE TO EXTERNAL EVENTS WHEN AWAKE
MOTOR STRENGTH PRESENT WHEN AROUSED FROM SLEEP;
PAROXYSMAL DROPPING INTO SLEEP STATE;

EEG is NOT abnormal EXCEPT that REM SLEEP ATTACKS occur immediately following AWAKE STATE & are NOT preceded by NON-REM sleep:

→ **NARCOLEPSY**

EEG shows NORMAL SLEEP PATTERN & WAKE CYCLES: 14 cps sleep spindles, esp. ant. head + sleep sharp-wave phase reversals @ vertex +/- k-complex on arousal: symmetric & diffuse series of fast waves (2-4 cps) = light sleep or 50% slow-wave activity with inc. amplitude & dec. frequency, esp. parietal = sleep humping: entire record diffuse high amplitude slow activity (0-4 cps DELTA) waves of deep sleep

→ **NORMAL SLEEP**

I. **NORMAL 1st STAGE SLEEP**: Eyes closed; pupils myotic; POSTURAL TONUS; EEG shows spindles & slow waves:

II. **PARADOXIC SLEEP**: cortical activity similar to WAKING + ABSENCE of electromyographic activity + muscular activity of the neck.
   A. **TONIC ACTIVITY**: for several minutes, accompanied by phasic behavioral & electrical phenomena;
      EEG: fast, low-voltage cortex - similar to waking; + regular THETA in HIPPOCAMPUS;
      EMG: absent activity.
   B. **PHASIC ACTIVITY**: **REM**: 50-60/minute; associated with CORTICAL & SUB-CORTICAL "PONTOGENICULO-OCCIPITAL ACTIVITY" (OR DEEP SLEEP WAVES).

2ND STAGE SLEEP: NON-REM HIGH VOLTAGE, RECORDED FROM RETICULAR FORMATION OF PONS & LATERAL GENICULATE OCCIPITAL CORTEX; IDENTICAL TO THAT RECORDED DURING VISUAL ATTENTION.

Ch. 3: EXAMINATIONS

Psychiatric Assessment

Name:	DOB:	Age:	Sex:
Appt Date:	Appt Start Time:		Appt End Time:
Provider:		People Present:	

Note Summary:

Last weight: Current weight: Height:

Review of Systems

Psychiatric:	Genitourinary:
Eyes:	Musculoskeletal:
Ear/Nose/Mouth/Throat:	Neurologic:
Cardiovascular:	Constitutional:
Endocrine:	Skin/Integument:
Respiratory:	Hematologic-lymphatic:
Gastrointestinal:	Allergic/Immunologic:

Mental Status Exam

General Appearance:	Thought Process:
Alertness:	Thought Content:
Eye Contact:	Perception:
Motor:	Orientation:
Gate/Station:	Concentration:
Affect:	Memory:
Mood:	Intellect:
Speech:	Insight:
Attitude:	Judgment:
Suicidal Ideation:	Fund of Knowledge:
Homicidal:	

Medication History

THOUGHT FORM (**CHECKLIST FOR "FORMAL THOUGHT DISORDER"**)

____ Incoherence (statements are incomprehensible)

____ Neologisms (made-up words)

____ Derailment (loose associations)

____ Poverty of Content (speaking platitudes, very sparse or "empty" conversations)

____ Illogicality (facts are obscured or distorted)

____ Perseveration (repeats same sentences over & over)

____ Blocking (long pauses between statements)

____ Concrete thinking (inability to derive abstract ideas from examples)

____ Thought insertion

____ Thoughts "taken away" from one's mind

____ Thought "diffusion" (seeming to be all around in the room)

____ Thought control (by outside source)

CHECKLIST FOR: LONG-TERM MEMORY

Ck (√) if Correct	PRESIDENTS NAMED BACKWARDS	OR NAMED FORWARD
☐	DONALD TRUMP	
☐	BARACK OBAMA	GEORGE WASHINGTON
☐	GEORGE W. BUSH	JOHN ADAMS
☐	BILL CLINTON	THOMAS JEFFERSON
☐	GEORGE H.W. BUSH	JAMES MADISON
☐	RONALD REAGAN	JAMES MONROE
☐	JIMMY CARTER	JOHN QUINCY ADAMS
☐	GERALD FORD	ANDREW JACKSON
☐	RICHARD NIXON	MARTIN VAN BUREN
☐	LYNDON B. JOHNSON	WILLIAM HENRY HARRISON
☐	JOHN F. KENNEDY	JOHN TYLER
☐	DWIGHT D. EISENHOWER	JAMES K. POLK
☐	HARRY S. TRUMAN	ZACHARY TAYLOR
☐	FRANKLYN D. ROOSEVELT	MILLARD FILLMORE
☐	HERBERT HOOVER	FRANKLIN PIERCE
☐	CALVIN COOLIDGE	JAMES BUCHANAN
☐	WARREN G. HARDING	ABRAHAM LINCOLN
☐	WOODROW WILSON	ANDREW JOHNSON
☐	WILLIAM HOWARD TAFT	ULYSSES S. GRANT
☐	THEODORE ROOSEVELT	RUTHERFORD B. HAYES
☐	WILLIAM McKINLEY	JAMES A. GARFIELD
☐	GROVER CLEVELAND	CHESTER A. ARTHUR

NAME:_____   DATE:_____

TEST FOR ABSTRACT THINKING   ABSTRACT CONCRETE LOGICAL AUTISTIC
                                    2 PTS.   1 PT.   2 PT   0

1. PEOPLE IN GLASS HOUSES SHOULDN'T THROW STONES.

2. EVERY CLOUD HAS A SILVER LINING.

3. A STITCH IN TIME SAVES NINE.

4. A PENNY SAVED IS A PENNY EARNED.

5. A BIRD IN THE HAND IS WORTH TWO IN THE BUSH.

6. YOU CAN'T JUDGE A BOOK BY ITS COVER.

7. HE WHO LAUGHS LAST, LAUGHS BEST.

8. DON'T PUT ALL YOUR EGGS IN ONE BASKET.

9. STILL WATER RUNS DEEP.

10. A ROLLING STONE GATHERS NO MOSS

                                   SUBTOTAL:

SET TEST:

1. FLOWERS:

2. ANIMALS:

3. COLORS:

4. TOWNS:

MENTAL STATUS EXAMINATION

General Appearance:

Attitude & Behavior:
Mood & Affect:

THOUGHT CONTENT	Hallucination						
	Delusion				Homicidality		Suicidal
THOUGHT PROCESS	COHERENT		LINEAR				OTHER:
ORIENT-ATION	Name		Date		Place		Circum-stance

MENTAL AGE

MEMORY								
	Immediate					5 digits	foreward	7.4 years
						4 digits	backward	9.5 years
						5 digits	backward	12.5 yrs
	Intermediate	Reduced	recall: only	___ words	OF 3 @ 5	MINUTES		
	Remote	>25%words	forgotten of	10 WORDS	TAUGHT X5	after 30 min	delay = 60'	_____
With Help		# WORDS	RECALLED	IF HINTS	GIVEN @	60 MINUTE	TESTING	_____
	SET TEST	SEMANTIC	MEMORY	10 **Fruits,**	10 **Animals,**	10 **Colors,**	10 **Towns**	_>29

FUND OF KNOW-LEDGE	President			Governor:			
	States Bordering						
							_____
							_____

PERCEPTUAL	VMI Clock:		popular pull			Roberts-2	_____
ATTENTION	Auditory	Attention	Span for	unrelated	words		
ABSTRACT THINKING	Proverb #1						
	Proverb #2						_____
	Sage Test	similarities					_____
CONCEN-TRATION	"DLROW"		spell world	backwards		Serial 7	subtraction	4.7 years
	"I am done"		2-Step COMMAND				3-Step COMMAND	_____
	interpersonal	challenges					
Persistence		Remember	a movie		a magazine		Hobbies
UseComputer							

INSIGHT		impairments	how it disables			
JUDGMENT	fire/theatre		pay by ck		why rules?	

EXPRESSIVE	**LANGUAGE**					
Reading						
Math						_____
Writing						

SCREENING TEST IQ		
FUNCTION ASSESSMENT	ADL timely	
ARTICULATION & MEMORY	20 syllable sentence	THE QUICK, BROWN FOX JUMPED OVER THE PICKET FENCE, THEN WENT ON HIS WAY WITHOUT STOPPING.
FUTURE PLANS?		

10 yrs

Mental Status Evaluation Summary

NAME: _____ D.O.B. _____

MANIC
____ Increased energy/drive/interests/ or psychomotor agitation;
____ Excessive pleasure-seeking behavior +/-painful consequences;
____ Long period of elevated/expansive or irritable mood;
____ Pressured speech/talkative with flight of ideas/racing thoughts;
____ Decreased need for sleep;
____ Inflated self-esteem/grandiosity;
____ Distracted by every stimulus.

ANXIETY
____ Trembling, twitching or feeling shaky
____ Muscle tension aches/soreness
____ Restlessness
____ Easy fatigability
____ Shortness of breath/smothering
____ Palpitations/inc. heart rate
____ Sweating/cold, clammy hands
____ Dry mouth
____ Dizziness/lightheadedness
____ Nausea/diarrhea/other GI distress
____ Flushes (hot flashes) or chills
____ Frequent urination
____ Dysphagia/"lump in throat"
____ Feeling keyed up or on edge
____ Exaggerated startle response
____ Difficulty concentrating/"going blank
____ Trouble falling/staying asleep
____ Irritability

DEPRESSION
____ Insomnia/hypersomnia almost daily;
____ Psychomotor retardation/agitation;
____ Feeling worthless/excessive guilt;
____ Impaired concentration/indecisive;
____ Depressed/irritable mood most of day;

DEMENTIA
____ Increasingly forgetful;
____ Impaired intermediate-memory;
____ Set Test score less than 29.
____ Impaired visuomotor integration.
____ Conceptual disorganization;
____ Concrete thinking.
____ Paucity of ideation.

PSYCHOTIC FEATURES
____ Grtr. than 30% loss global function on GAF without organic cause;
____ Loss of drive & interests;
____ Extreme social withdrawl;
____ Affect flat/ or abnormal to ideation;
____ Marked decreased concern for personal hygiene or grooming;
____ Poverty of speech content;
____ Derailment; continuous illogic. speech;
____ Hallucinations; audio ___ vis ___ tact ___
____ Delusions: mood congruent; ___
____ mood incongruent; paranoid; ___
____ thought-broadcasting; control;
influence ___; reference ___;
thought insertion ___ or deletion ___;
____ Assaultive; (or dangerous)
____ Suicidal attempt;

ASSESSMENT OF CAPACITY
____ Lacks understanding of the problem;
____ Cannot communicate his/her needs;
____ Lacks appropriate goals or wishes;
____ I.Q. measured below 70.

DELIRIUM
____ Disoriented;
____ Altered level of consciousness;
____ Extreme hypervigilance or somnolence;
____ Extremely short attention span;
____ Extremely distractible or unarousable;
____ Pupillary abnormalities; Blurred vision/dry skin or clammy skin;
____ Fever/tachycardia/bradycardial abn. BP;
____ Abnormal neurological reflexes;
____ Extreme emotional lability;
____ Disinhibited or intrusive;
____ Perseverative; Personal or safety neglect;
____ Abnormal speech;
____ History of drug intake/abuse.

SCHIZOPHRENIC RESIDUALS
____ Illogical interpretation of proverbs;
____ Autistic conceptualizations.
____ Blunted affect

DATE: _____ SIGNATURE: _____

Test for AUDITORY ATTENTION SPAN

Client:
Date:
CA:
MA:
ATTENTION QUOTIENT:

dog axe						
cat west						
ear fence	song					
boat night	clock					
key mud	oats coat					
pig vase	tub road					
ice dress	knob ten plant					
ink rain	friends stone ship					
freeze chair	horse pipe milk shoe					
rope cross	toad north skirt mule					
lamp hair	fan spend skate flour	east				
wool cart	fish barn desk blot	toad				
	64 = 17-0 65 = 17-6	66 = 18-0 67 = 18-6	68 = 18-9 69 = 19-0			
	54 = 12-0 55 = 12-6	57 = 13-6 58 = 14-0	59 = 14-6 60 = 15-0	61 = 15-6	62 = 16-0 63 = 16-6	
	45 = 8-3 46 = 8-6	47 = 9-0 48 = 9-6	49 = 10-0 50 = 10-3	51 = 10-9	52 = 11-0 53 = 11-6	
	36 = 5-6 37 = 5-9	38 = 6-0 39 = 6-3	40 = 6-9 41 = 7-3	42 = 7-6	43 = 7-9 44 = 8-0	
SCORING:	27 = 3-0 28 = 3-3	29 = 3-6 30 = 3-9	31 = 4-0 32 = 4-3	33 = 4-6	34 = 4-9 35 = 5-0	

Intermediate Memory Testing

HOW TO USE: After I say these 10 words, please immediately REPEAT THEM. I will TEACH THEM TO YOU EVERY 5 MINUTES, 4 MORE TIMES. REMEMBER THEM.

RECALL

IMMEDIATE	
5 MINUTE RECALL	
10 MINUTE RECALL	
15 MINUTE RECALL	
45 MINUTE RECALL	
1 HOUR RECALL	
FAILURE IS <50%%	

RECENT/ INTERMEDIATE MEMORY TESTING

WORDS TO REMEMBER	Immediate	5 MINUTES	10 MINUTES	15 MINUTES	45 MINUTES
DOG					
AXE					
WEST					
EAR					
FENCE					
SONG					
BOAT					
NIGHT					
CLOCK					
KEY					
TOTAL					

NEUROLOGICAL EXAMINATION: _____

Cranial Nerves: I Smell Right ___ Left ___;   II Vision Ck: Right ___ Left ___
Visual Fields Intact: Left ___ Right ___   Fundoscopic Exam: Right ___ Left ___
III, IV, VI Pupils   Left: ___ Left: ___   Extraocular Motion: Right ___ Left ___
V Jaw Movement: ___ Sensation ___   Corneal Reflex: Right ___ Left ___
VII Facial Weakness: Voluntary _____   Reflex Movements   Right ___ Left ___
VIII Whisper Heard Right ___ Left ___   Tuning Forks: _____
IX; X Palate no deviation ___ Gag intact ___ Pharynx sensation   Right ___ Left ___
XI Sternomastoid Shrug _____   Strength   Right ___ Left ___
XII Tongue   protrudes midline ___ no atrophy ___ no fasciculation's _____
Speaks without dysarthria _____

Reflexes: Bic. Tri. Br. R. Hoff. Pat. Act. Bab.   Other Abd. Crem. Anal
Right: ___   ___   ___   ___   ___   ___   ___   ___   ___   ___   ___
Left: ___   ___   ___   ___   ___   ___   ___   ___   ___   ___   ___

Gait & Station: _____

Motor System:
Strength/ Atrophy: _____
Fasciculations: _____
Tone/ Spasticity: _____
Involuntary Movements: _____
Tremor / Rigidity: _____
Hypokinesia: _____
Movement / Hopping: _____
Associated Movements: _____
Ataxia: F-N H-S: _____
Alternating Movements: _____
Diadokokinesis: _____
Drift / Rebound: _____
Trophic Changes: _____
Horner's: _____
Vaso-sudomotor: _____
Sphincters: _____
Respiratory: _____

Sensory System:
Touch/2-Point: _____ Pain: _____ Thermal: _____
Position / Vibration: _____
Romberg / Deep Pain: _____
Paresthesia: _____ Double Stimulation: _____ Causalgia: _____
Subjective Pain: _____
Stereognosia: _____

CRANIAL NERVE EXAMINATION

I Olfactory: ____ peppermint; ____ coffee; ____ cinnamon; ____ other

II Optic:
Fundoscopic:_____

visual fields:_____

far vision _____ near vision

III Oculomotor; IV Trochlear; VI Abducens: pupils round ____; equal ____; reactive to light ____ & accommodation ____
normal voluntary gaze in all directions _____ without diplopia; ____ without nystagmus; other _____

V Trigeminal: corneal reflex intact on R ____; L ____; sensitivity anterior 2/3 tongue ____; sensitivity of Trigeminal I ____; II____; III ____
jaw reflex +1, +2, +3, +4, +5.
_____

VII Facial: raises eyebrows ____; closes eyes tight ____; smiles with eyes closed; symmetrically ____; puffs cheeks R____; L ____

VIII Acoustic: hearing 2048 hz ____; R ____; L ____ Rinne: AC > BC
sound localization   R____; L ____

IX Vagus & X Glossopharyngeal: posterior pharynx sensitive on R ____ L____; uvula midline ____; gag reflex intact ____

XI Sternocleidomastoid: turns head to right ____; turns head to left ____; shrugs shoulders bilaterally ____

XII Hypoglossal: normal tongue protrusion ____; strong push against right cheek ____; left cheek ____. Can say "Methodist Episcopal" ____

Meningeal Signs: the neck is supple ____.

NEUROLOGICAL EXAMINATION: CRANIAL NERVES
_____
                                        patient   date

I. ____ cannot smell __vanilla, __lemon, __tobacco, __coffee, __mint.

II. ____ Abnormal visual acuity: ___Snellen: ___other. R 20/___ L 20/___

    ____ Abnormal Visual Fields Exam: ___tangent screen: ___perimetry: ___confront.
    ____ "cortical blindness" on double simultaneous stimulation of visual field.

    OS   first   OD
                                      test
                                      each
                                      eye
         A   B   separ-   C   D
                                      ately:
                                      then
                                      use
                                      bilateral
                                      stimulation

    ____ Blink reflex lost (object approaching blind eye not perceived).
    ____ Optokinetic nystagmus lost when following rotating drum.
    ____ Light reflex direct   lost: R ____ : L ____

    ____ Abnormal fundoscopic exam:

    OD   OS

    ____ retinal pigmentation abnormally increased: /____ decreased.
    ____ retinal cherry red spot.

    ____ optic disc margin blurred: "choked disc":
         ___Pseudopapilledema = excessive glial proliferation at disc margin:
            venous pulsations present: normal blind spot: no inc. IC pressure.
         ___Papillitis (optic neuropathy): extensive visual field defect early -
            especially central scotoma (may clear after 2 weeks) or blurred disc
            may progress to pallor & demyelination of optic nerve.
         ___Papilledema: minimal field defect initially: early stage = vascular
            congestion; capillary dilation with redness of discs; engorgement of
            veins ± absence of venous pulsations: late stage = small splinter
            hemorrhages in radial distribution; elevation of disc margins with
            tortuous & distended overlying vessels & multiple hemorrhages:
            chronic stage = gliotic changes obscuring details over nerve head;
            decrease of vascular distention & hemorrhages; enlargement of blind
            spot & peripheral constriction of visual field: papilledema usually
            associated with increased intracranial pressure.

CRANIAL NERVES:

		patient			date
		Shape	Size in mm.	Light reflex	Accomodation Reflex
____	PUPIL ABNORMAL:				
	Right eye = OD				
	Left eye = OS				

Code for reflex
+ = active reflex
± = sluggish
0 = non-reactive

____ EXCURSION TEST ABNORMAL for 6 cardinal positions of gaze on __R: __L eye.

```
    III. ↑ superior rectus          III. ↑ inferior oblique     superior rectus ↑ III.
    VI.          III.                    III.                              VI.
←  lat. rectus  med. rectus →       ←  med. rectus                       lat. rectus →
         OD                                              OS
    III. ↓ inferior rectus         IV. ↓ superior oblique    inferior rectus ↓ III.
```

____ COVER TEST ABNORMAL: patient fixates on distant object; one eye is covered while other is observed for movement (or deviation).
Primary deviation = the deflection of the strabismic eye in the direction opposite to the normal action of the paralyzed muscle (while eyes look in field of action of paralyzed muscle).
Secondary deviation = the deflection of the normal eye when covered - while the affected eye fixes on an object.

____ LATENT STRABISMUS: (HETEROPHORIA)
  __both eyes normal when uncovered: no deviation at rest position.
  __cover test abnormal: when one eye is covered, it deviates & returns to original position when screen is removed.

____ NON-PARALYTIC STRABISMUS:
  __deviation of eyes present in rest position.
  __normal range of motion for each eye on excursion test: deviation equal for all positions of gaze.
  __cover test: secondary and primary deviations are equal.

____ PARALYTIC STRABISMUS: (OPHTHALMOPLEGIA)
  __eyes usually not deviated in rest position.
  __excursion test shows limitation of movement of eye in the field of action of the paralyzed muscle only.
  __cover test: secondary deviation greater than primary deviation.
  __false projection present: closing patient's sound eye as he quickly points to object in front of him - his finger is directed to the side of the object corresponding to the field of action of the paralyzed muscle.
  __diplopia present initially at least.
  __ataxic gait, head tilt & vertigo may be present.

III. ____ ptosis: inability to open eyelid.
     ____ pupil dilated
     ____ direct pupil light reflex absent: consensual light reflex absent.
     ____ direct blink reflex absent: consensual blink reflex present.
     ____ inability to move eye upward, inward & downward (from lateral position).
     ____ eye turned outward (laterally) & downward.
     ____ diplopia present.

NEUROLOGICAL EXAMINATION: CRANIAL NERVES

                                                          patient   date

IV. ____ eye fails to move downward (especially when turned medially).
     ____ diplopia (in vertical plane).

VI. ____ lateral eye movement weakness/paralysis.
     ____ diplopia on lateral gaze (if acute).

V. ____ corneal reflex lost.
    ____ loss of pain & touch over frontal scalp, above eyes; above lips & over cheeks & chin.
    ____ loss of taste of salt & vinegar, anterior tongue.
    ____ weak masseter & temporal muscles on teeth clenching.
    ____ weak pterygoids on pressing jaw against examiner's finger (mouth open).
    ____ masseter paralysis/weakness: opening mouth causes deviation of jaw to weak side
    ____ atrophy of masseter, temporalis or pterygoids.
    ____ fasciculations of masseter, temporalis or pterygoids.

VII. ____ (Parotid branch): cannot whistle
      ____ (Parotid branch): mouth drawn to sound side; sags on affected side.
      ____ (Parotid branch): cannot wrinkle forehead (infranuclear -orbicularis oculi).
      ____ (Parotid branch): cannot close eye: palpebral fissure widened.

      ____ (Chorda tympani): loss of taste - ipselateral 2/3 tongue anteriorly.

      ____ defect lacrimation & salivation (parasympathetic division).

      ____ (Supranuclear): contralateral weakness mouth with ability to wrinkle forehead retained: flattening of nasolabial fold & weakness retracting corner of mouth.

VIII. ____ loss of auriculopalpebral (startle) reflex.
       ____ Weber test (tuning fork mid-forehead) shows deafness on one side: _R: _L.
       ____ Rinne test shows conductive loss: air conduction <u>less</u> than bone conduction
       ____ Audiometry abnormal:

	2000 cps			4000 cps	
0 = normal	R 25 db	45 db	R	25 db	45 db
X = abnormal	L 25 db	45 db	L	25 db	45 db

       ____ Nylen-Barany test reproduces vertigo attack (going from sitting to supine with head dropped 45° over table edge).
       ____ Barany Rotation Test produces vertigo (10 rotations within 20 seconds).
       ____ Sudden turning when walking produces vertigo.
       ____ Nystagmus present: horizontal, vertical or with a rotatory component.
       ____ Oscillopsia present (feeling the environment is moving in one direction: illusory movement during the slow involuntary phase of nystagmus).
       ____ Ice caloric test abnormal: (normal = tonic deviation to same side & clonic or quick phase nystagmus to opposite side).
       ____ Warm caloric test abnormal: (normal = tonic deviation to opposite side & clonic quick phase to same side which is stimulated with warm water).

DESCRIBE NYSTAGMUS: _____

CRANIAL NERVES: _____
                           patient   date

IX. _____ loss of taste on posterior 1/3 tongue.
    _____ sensory deficit on palate & pharynx.
    _____ pain in throat on swallowing (glossopharyngeal neuralgia).
    _____ weakness of elevation & abduction of pharyngeal wall (stylopharyngeus
          muscle weakness).

X. _____ dysphonia: difficulty with phonation: abductor paralysis of vocal cord:
          __hoarseness (unilateral paralysis):
          __aphonia (loss of voice); dyspnea; stridor (bilateral paralysis).
    _____ dysphagia: weakness or paralysis of swallowing: weakness or paralysis of
          soft palate which sags: involvement of muscles of deglutition if nucleus
          ambiguuous involved with weakness of middle & inferior constrictors of
          pharynx: regurgitation of food through the nose (inability to close
          pharynx when swallowing): weakness or loss of movement of "Adam's apple"
          when swallowing.
    _____ loss of palatal-pharyngeal "gag" reflex.
    _____ sensory deficit external auditory meatus & ear pinna.

XI. _____ flatness of neck on paralyzed side: rotation of neck does not reveal
          sternocleidomastoid muscle body.
    _____ weak head flexion upon neck (if bilateral paralysis).
    _____ trapezius paralysis: weakness of shoulder-shrugging & in raising arm above
          horizontal plane: there may be slight winging of scapula with atrophy &
          flattening of neck region

XII. _____ tongue weakness: on pressing tip of tongue against cheek (mild deficit) or
           on tongue protrusion (severe deficit).
     __deviation of tongue to affected side (e.g. side of hemiplegia): no
       atrophy or fasciculations (upper motor neuron XII lesion).
     __indentations or scalloping along tongue edges or gross atrophy &
       fasciculations of tongue (lower motor neuron XII lesion).
     __positive tensilon test (Myasthenia gravis only).

A.R. = against resistance

NEUROMUSCULAR EXAMINATION

0 = no contraction
1 = trace
2 = active movement if gravity eliminated
3 = active movement against gravity
4 = active movement against gravity & resistance
5 = normal power

NECK: flex, extend, rotate	Deep neck muscles	cervical	C1-4
SHOULDER: shrug A.C.	Trapezius	Accessory	C3,4
Shoulder: medial adduction & elevate	Rhomboids	Dors. Scapular	C4,5
ARMS: (raised) adducting A.R.	Pectoralis Major	Lat. & M. Pect.	C5-8
ARMS: abducting A.R.	Supraspinatus	Suprascapular	C5
ARMS: flex supinated arm A.R.	Biceps	Musculocutaneous	C5-6
ARMS: abduction maintained A.R.	Deltoid	Circumflex	C5,6
ARMS: adduct (horiz. extended) A.R.	Latissimus Dorsi	N. to Lat. Dorsi	C6-8
ARMS: extend forearm A.R.	Triceps	Radial	C6-8
FOREARM: (between P & S) flex A.R.	Brachioradialis	Radial	C5,6
FOREARM: (arm e)resist hand pronation	Supinator	Radial	C5,6
WRIST: (fingers ext.)ext. wrist radially	Ext. Carp. Rad.	Radial	C6,7
FINGERS: extension A.R.	Ext. Digitorum	Radial	C7,8
WRIST: extend A.R. towards ulnar	Ext. Carp. Ulnaris	Radial	C7,8
ARM: (extended) resist supination	Pronator Teres	Median	C6,7
WRIST: flex fist A.R. toward radial	Flexor Carpi Radial	Median	C6,7,8
FINGERS: flex		Median	C6-T1
HIP: (knee f. -leg support) flex AR	Iliopsoas	Femoral	L1,2,3
HIP: (lat. rotated) flex knee A.R.	Sartorius	Femoral	L2,3
LEG: extend A.R.	Quadriceps	Femoral	L2-4
LEG: adduct A.R.	Adductors	Obturator	L2-4
LEG: (prone)lift knee from table AR	Glut. Maximus	Inferior Gluteal	L5,S1-2
HIP: int. rotation (knee flex)lateral move	(Glut med & min)	Superior Gluteal	L4,5; S1
LEG: abduction (sup. leg ext) A.R.	Tensor Fascia Lata)	"	"
LEG: flex A.R. (prone)	Hamstring(med.= semitendinosis)Sciatic		L4-S1
	(lat = biceps femoris)		
LEG: plantarflex ankle A.R.	Gastrocnemius	Sciatic	S1,2
FOOT: (prone) invert flexed foot AR	Tibialis Posterior	Scalar	L4,5
FOOT: evert A.R.	Peroneus long/brev	Sciatic	L5,S1
FOOT: dorsiflex ankle AR	Tibialis Anterior	Sciatic	L5,S1
FOOT: dorsiflex toes A.R.	Ext. Dig. Longus	Sciatic	L5,S1
TOE: dorsiflex great toe A.R.	Ext. Hallu Longus	Sciatic	L5,S1
	Ext. Digitorum Brev	Sciatic	S1

CHAPTER 3: EXAMINATIONS

After reviewing the Neurocognitive Questionnaire, Diagnostics, Health History/ Review of Systems, Neurological Examination and physical findings, a meticulous **Mental Status Examination** should be performed. Getting the "gestalt" of the patient's **General Appearance** screens for physical illness sometimes as well as for **neglect** (of hygiene/ cleanliness/ grooming/ dressing/, etc.). Unless caused by physical disability, this is often seen in the dementias or in severe depression (especially with psychotic features) as well as in delirium and severe bipolar mania.

Sensing a patient's **Attitude** and **Behavior** is also very helpful in diagnosis. There may be extreme boastfulness or grandiosity (often seen in the manic state of a bipolar disorder) or there may appear a sense of overwhelming defeat or loss (often seen in Major Depressive Disorder). There may be a sense of "edginess" or of being "keyed-up" (often seen in anxiety states). Or else the unusual look of detachment (between the patient's feelings and expressed language) may suggest schizophrenia, or possibly Autism Spectrum Disorder. Delirious patients usually show a **disorder of arousal** - whether the disinhibition of impulsivity or else the lethargy and somnolence (sometimes slipping into coma).

Mood (how a patient feels), and **Affect** (the emotions observed by the clinician) are critical. Facial expressions are often helpful. A depressed patient usually appears empty, sad and bleak. Schizophrenics often present with apathy and a vacant stare - avoiding eye contact - and showing a paucity of facial expressions. Anxious patients look more "keyed-up" and may have been "biting their fingernails". Facial expressions in dementia vary with the stage of illness. In early dementia patients appear frustrated and ashamed of their slipping capacities. In later stage dementia, patients may puzzle the clinician in appearance with their blatant denial of their incapacities. Very late stage dementia shows overwhelming incapacity and problems with ambulation, bowel and bladder control, etc.

Memory evaluation usually comes next. However, it is suggested that on arrival for the examination, some sort of beginning to the process introduce initially the **Intermediate Memory Test** of the "10 Words" (see p. 81) Then, every 5 minutes for 3 additional occasions during the mental status examination, ask the patient to say the words again (record the answers) and **re-teach** the missing words. This allows a 45 minute to 1 hour "final examination" which can be substituted as a **Remote Memory Test.** Asking the patient to name the presidents forward or backwards is occasionally used to assess remote memory or general information during a patient's lifetime - as is asking the patient to name the governor, and bordering states of the patient's home state. The primary disorder of **delirium** is impairment in **Immediate Memory & Attention**. This can often be tested with digit span memory. Failure to repeat 5 digits forward and 4 digits backwards shows more than a 50% loss of this capacity. The Detroit Test for Auditory Attention Span for Unrelated Words is a much more accurate way of getting age equivalents for the total number of words recalled - but this is a more time-consuming test. When checking for sustained attention and concentration, the clinician asks the patient to "spell *'world'* backwards" - or "subtract 7 from 100 and continue subtracting 7 from the answer for at least 4 more times". The patient is then asked to "follow a 3-step command" such as (1) "Take this paper with your right hand;" (2) "Fold the paper if half"; and (3) "Give it back to me with your left hand". A five-year-old child can usually perform a 3-step command successfully but a delirious patient often finds this difficult.

Memory examination is critical for discriminating schizophrenia, Autism Spectrum Disorder, and Anxiety Disorders (which **do not** typically show memory impairment) from the other neurocognitive disorders (which usually **are** characterized by progressive loss of intermediate memory (e.g., in amnestic disorders) and especially loss of remote memory over time (as seen in the dementias). The **limbic** system (which consists of the hippocampus, thalamus, hypothalamus, basal ganglia and cingulate gyrus) is critical for "making and retrieving memories". So once this is injured (as in "Amnestic Disorders") there may be a loss of memory storage from that time: this is called "anterograde amnesia". It will manifest sometime later as a "remote memory loss". This remote memory impairment is more easily tested by asking the patient to describe his memorable events "over the past 2 years" (or since any known traumatic event).

Neurologists, such as Raymond Adams, have described such distinctions as "Axial Amnesia" (as exemplified by the alcoholic Korsakoff's Psychosis) involving predominantly the limbic system of the brain - - - as opposed to "Cortical Amnesia" (as exemplified by Alzheimer's Disease) - - - involving focal deficits of the cerebral cortex. It is probably more useful to differentiate the memory functions as (1) **IMMEDIATE**: SHORT-TERM MEMORY/ **ATTENTION DISORDERS** stemming from the brain's **Reticular Activating System** (as exemplified by **delirium**); (2) **INTERMEDIATE / RECENT MEMORY DISORDERS** stemming from the **Limbic Region** of the brain (and as exemplified by limbic encephalitis, concussion, and other **amnestic states**); and (3) **REMOTE / LONG-TERM MEMORY DISORDERS** stemming from focal cortical deficits such as senile plaques of amyloid, or tau protein accumulations with neurofibrillary tangles in brain cortical foci (exemplified by Alzheimer's Disease). As previously stated, initial damage to the hippocampus may be responsible for the subsequent inability to store memories and retrieve stored memories after a time lapse. Luria's "10 Word Test" is useful for testing for the intermediate memory impairment component. And "long-term" memory can be screened by asking for the words recalled at 45 minutes or 1 hour (i.e., the end of a typical Mental Status Examination). Additionally, it has been shown that Alzheimer's Disease patients rarely are helped when "hints" are given for the words (see p. 141) whereas Lewy Body Dementia (and usually Parkinson's Disease Dementia often improve their scores when the hints are given (see LONG TERM MEMORY TESTING at the end of **Chapter 6**).

The clinician examines **Thought Process** looking for slowness of thinking or speaking as seen in delirium with lethargy, and in dementia as well as severe depression and schizophrenia. Processing speed may be accelerated in anxiety and in Bipolar manic states (as well as in delirium caused by stimulants). The clinician is also checking for **coherence** of speech which is often absent in schizophrenia, delirium and late stage dementia. Absence of connectedness in communication or **linearity** of speech suggests schizophrenia which often shows a classic sign of **derailment** or what has been termed *alusive thinking* - where the initial subject and predicate seem to have no understandable relationship to the remaining "tail of the sentence" - and yet the **flow** of the sentence or "prosody" is seamless. Only schizophrenics appear capable of such language; whereas bipolar patients, esp. in manic states are frequently noted to show a "flight of ideas" and "tangentiality" where many subjects and their predicates flow freely yet **don't seem to be "sequential"** but are rather a rapid change of topics. (There is an **illogical** aspect to the *allusive derailment* of schizophrenia). Additionally, **concrete thinking** is often seen in schizophrenia (e.g. on the "Proverbs Test" for abstract thinking) but it is a signature impairment of mental immaturity and dementia as well. **Conceptual disorganization** is more a signature impairment of schizophrenia (which is excluded currently from the neurocognitive disorders) and it is present in many neurocognitive disorders such as delirium, Korsakoff's syndrome, and late dementia, etc.

One also examines **Thought Content** to rule out auditory hallucinations which are interpreted as coming from **outside the head** when found in "functional" or "organic" conditions. Schizophrenics especially are notable for "hearing two separate voices which comment continuously on the patient's behavior". Sometimes they are actually welcomed as "good company"; sometimes they are frightening. There may be visual hallucinations as well. Schizophrenics are more apt to suffer with visions of "frightening faces" (especially in paranoia) whereas in organic psychoses such as in epilepsy or brain tumors, the visual imperceptions may take the form of "colors and shapes". Sensory/ tactile hallucinations may be experienced in all these illnesses. But olfactory hallucinations (experiencing strange or horrific smells) are again more commonly found in "organic" conditions such as seizure activity. When the tactile experience is "numbness" or tingling paresthesias, one should always seek a neurological condition such as diabetic neuropathy first.

Thought Content is also examined for items such as **delusions**. People with late stage dementia may suffer with delusions such as "the person living with them isn't really their spouse" or "someone is continuously hiding their keys or eyeglasses" - - - "trying to drive them crazy". Paranoid, fixed **complex delusional states** are almost always a sign of paranoid schizophrenia, however. A major usefulness for examining thought content is to rule out severe Major Depressive Disorder by checking for feelings of hopelessness, helplessness, uselessness and worthlessness - - - and especially by checking for a history of suicide attempts and recent suicidal ideation and plans. Bipolar, depressed patients, may admit a prior history of suicidality with intermittent "very productive" career periods (or dangerously high-risk energy states).

The MDQ (Mood Disorder Questionnaire) which is in the public domaine, is easily scored and is helpful in discriminating between a unipolar vs. a bipolar depressive state.

Of course, one must screen for homicidality as well. There has been a rash of "suicide by cops" lately where the perpetrator wants the police to kill the perpetrator while provoking the police with a "mass slaughter". Schizophrenics are blamed frequently for these events although the percentage of violence among the mentally ill is relatively low. Nevertheless, schizophrenics do show early **impairments of Judgment and Insight** into their illness and its consequences. These two cognitive functions are also progressively impaired in delirium and later stages of dementia.

Functional Capacity Assessment is very necessary in all the neurocognitive disorders. Many bipolars make high-salaried movie stars or financial magnates and only need help in the deteriorating stages of illness unfortunately. (Treatment in the early stages may prevent these dangerous stages).

The Group for the Advancement of Psychiatry (Barbara Long, M.D., Ph.D.; Andrew O. Brown, M.D.; with Sean-Sassano-Higgins, M.D.. & David "Daven" E. Morrison, MD) has published Functional assessment for Disability Applications to include:

1 SOCIAL COMPETENCE AND/OR TEAMWORK: can the person communicate, cooperate & cooperate with peers subordinates, or authority figures at the workplace;

2 ADAPTABILITY/ FLEXIBILITY: the ability to change one's perspective responding to changing demands.

3 CONSCIENTIOUSNESS/ DEPENDABILITY: reliabiity & consistency in performing one's duties.

4 IMPULSE & BEHAVIORAL CONTROL: is the individual's impulsivity likely to impair work capacity;

5 INTEGRITY: is the individual's trustworthiness sufficient to perform this specific work demand?

In assessing a patient for loss of/ impaired language capacities one makes note of the following:
1. Auditory Verbal Comprehension;
2. Word-Finding Ability;
3. Naming ability;
4. Automatic Speech;
5. Ability to Count from one to twenty;
6. Ability to remember the alphabet, days of the week & months of the year;

One might also ask the patient to "sing a song" such as "Twinkle, Twinkle, Little Star".

The clinician should also check for verbal apraxia for sentences - such as repeating a 20-syllable sentence: e.g., **"THE QUICK, BROWN FOX JUMPED OVER THE WHITE PICKET FENCE AND THEN WENT BRISKLY ON HIS WAY"**.

The clinician should then check for **non-verbal** praxis, e.g.:

___ "TOUCH YOUR EAR", ___ "NOSE"; ___ "LIPS"; ___ "HAIR".

___ " SHOW ME HOW YOU USE A HAMMER"; and

___ "PRETEND YOU ARE WAVING GOODBYE"

The "Clock-Setting" and "MAZE" escapes are also important parts of a complete Mental Status Examination. The "SET TEST" is useful for detecting late dementia where the patient cannot name (and score 1 point for each of) 10 **F**lowers; 10 **A**nimals; 10 **C**olors; and 10 **T**owns or cities (also called the **FACT** Test) - which tests for categorization ability. Scoring below 30 of the 40 points requested is often diagnostic of a dementia.

DIFFERENTIATING NEUROCOGNITIVE DISORDERS

FORGETTING names of acquaintances after brief separations; forgetting doctor appointments & taking one's medications; misplacing things; difficulty organizing tasks; getting lost in familiar places

FAILS SHORT-TERM MEMORY ("ATTENTION") TEST

DRAW: Blood Tests for HYPERCOAGULATION PROFILE; & TSH, Free T4, T3, Thyroid peroxidase antibodies & antithyroglobulin; & as indicated HIV, CNS fungus (aspergillosis); VDRL for syphilis; Lyme disease; Balumuthia/ Whipple's Disease: ELECTROLYTES (Sodium, Potassium, Calcium/Magnesium/ Phosphate; Chloride; Bicarbonate; & Albumin; 17-OHCS & 17-KS; Blood Gases; Serum Ammonia ,Acetone & Cholesterol, & Alpha2Globulins; Plasma Creatinine; Renin; Aldosterone; VITAMIN B1,B12/cyancobalamine; niacin/folate; BUN; U/A ketones, glucose, pH, protein; ammonia; oxalate crystals; HEAVY METAL screen; ANA titer. ORDER Brain Angiogram; Echocardiogram; Carotid Ultra

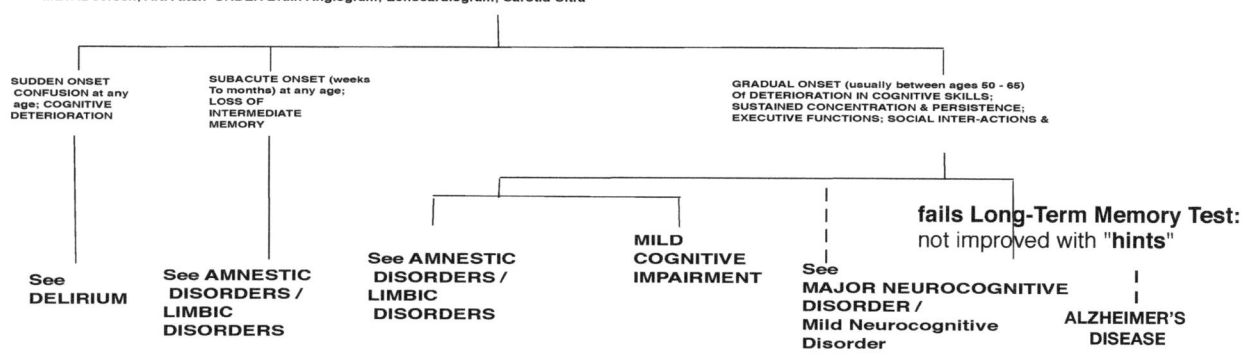

- **SUDDEN ONSET CONFUSION** at any age; COGNITIVE DETERIORATION
  - See **DELIRIUM**

- **SUBACUTE ONSET** (weeks To months) at any age; LOSS OF INTERMEDIATE MEMORY
  - See **AMNESTIC DISORDERS / LIMBIC DISORDERS**

- **GRADUAL ONSET** (usually between ages 50 – 65) Of DETERIORATION IN COGNITIVE SKILLS; SUSTAINED CONCENTRATION & PERSISTENCE; EXECUTIVE FUNCTIONS; SOCIAL INTER-ACTIONS &
  - See **AMNESTIC DISORDERS / LIMBIC DISORDERS**
  - **MILD COGNITIVE IMPAIRMENT**
  - See **MAJOR NEUROCOGNITIVE DISORDER / Mild Neurocognitive Disorder**
  - **fails Long-Term Memory Test:** not improved with "**hints**"
    - **ALZHEIMER'S DISEASE**

	ATTENTION & IMMEDIATE MEMORY primary memory	INTERMEDIATE MEMORY secondary memory	REMOTE MEMORY tertiary memory
CAPACITY	limited (7 ± 2 digits)	very large	probably unlimited
DURATION	seconds	minutes to years	may be permanent
ENTRY INTO STORAGE	verbal recording	rehearsal	overlearning
ACCESSIBILITY	very rapid	relatively slow	very rapid
TYPE OF INFORMATION	probably verbal	all	all
EFFECT OF DISTRACTION	labile	labile	stable
TYPE OF FORGETTING OR INFORMATION LOSS	new information replaces old	interference: retroactive & proactive inhibition	may be none
ANATOMIC SITES OF DYSFUNCTION	RETICULAR ACTIVATING SYSTEM	LIMBIC SYSTEM	ASSOCIATION CORTEX
CLINICAL TESTS	digit span Detroit test for Auditory Attention Span For Unrelated Words Vigilance Tasks	recall after distraction: Wechsler Delayed Logical Memory Test: Luria Learning Curve For Unrelated Words	WAIS General Information previously learned information & skill
CLINICAL EXAMPLES ONSET:	Acute:Delirium, "toxic psychosis"; "acute brain syndrome" ; encephalitis-opathy: Episodic: petit mal or psychomotor seizures Chronic: minimal cerebral dysfunction i.e., AD/HD	herpes limbic encephalopathy: Acute: anterior communicating artery aneurysm/infarct: remote effect of CA (prostate,ovaries,breast) Episodic: Basilar artery migraine; basilar artery transient ischemic attacks (T.I.A.)-vert.artery compression Transient: Posttraumatic amnesia: unilateral infarct left hippocampal region: thiamine deficit/Korsakoff's: Gradual: Korsakoff's Syndrome: brain tumor/abscess with bilateral medial temporal involvement/ colloid cyst 3rd v. Chronic course: any of above	Acute:pancreatitis: ICP / Occult Hydro Subacute: Jakob-Creutzfeld slow virus S.I.A.D.H.:autoimm polyarteritis; syph CNS A-V malformatic Hypothyroid; adrena insufficiency/Cushi Step-wise:Lacunar s of hypertensive CVA Binswanger's of sub cortical arterioscl otic leukoencephalo Gradual: (sloppy) Pick (neat) Alzheimer's: (after 65) Senile:

Ch. 4: DELIRIUM

DELIRIUM

Because the Neurocognitive Disorders have always been included in the five editions of the **Diagnostic and Statistical Manual of Mental Disorders**, including the 2022 **DSM-5-TR**, one might presume they are "mental", i.e., "functional" disorders. Nothing could be further from the truth!

Except for excluding some (1) Dissociative Disorders; (2) Major Depressive Disorders; and (3) Schizophrenic Disorders - all of which can present with *confusion syndromes*, the remaining diagnoses would best be considered to be *neurological disorders*. Many might be considered encephalopathies or even encephalitis - as will be seen below.

DSM-5-TR recognizes this fact in "Point 5":

> *"There is evidence from the history, physical examination or laboratory findings that the disturbance is a direct physiological consequence of another medical condition, substance intoxication or withdrawal (i.e., due to a drug abuse or to a medication) or exposure to a toxin or is due to multiple etiologies".* [See following 2 pages]

NEUROCOGNITIVE DISORDERS

SUDDEN ONSET of DETERIORATION in a person's **attention; memory; perception; cognitive speed;** or **behaviors** - which were previously acquired. This may have a **genetic etiology which can present any age.**

GRADUAL ONSET OF DETERIORATION IN a person's sustained concentration and persistence; executive functions; social interactions and adaptation capacity; understanding and memory

see **Major & Minor Neurocognitive Disorders**

DELIRIUM FROM SUBSTANCE USE

F10.221 ALCOHOL USE DISORDER
F10.231 ALCOHOL WITHDRAWL DISORDER
F12.221 CANNABIS USE DISORDER
F16.221 PHENCYCLIDINE USE DISORDER
F16.121 OTHER HALLUCINOGEN USE DISORDER
F18.221 INHALENT USE DISORDER
F11.221 OPOID USE DISORDER
F11.991 OPOID USE DISORDER (PRESCRIBED0
F13.221 SEDATIVE, HYPNOTIC, OR ANXIOLYTIC USE DISORDER
F15.221 AMPHETAMINE/ OTHER STIMULANT USE DISORDER
F15.921 AMPHETAMINE USE DISORDER (PRESCRIBED)
F14.221 COCAINE USE DISORDER
F19.221 OTHER (or UNKNOWN) USE DISORDER
F19.921 UNKNOWN PRESCRIBED MEDICATION USE

Substitute suffix .121 if mild use disorder

F41.0 UNSPECIFIED DELIRIUM

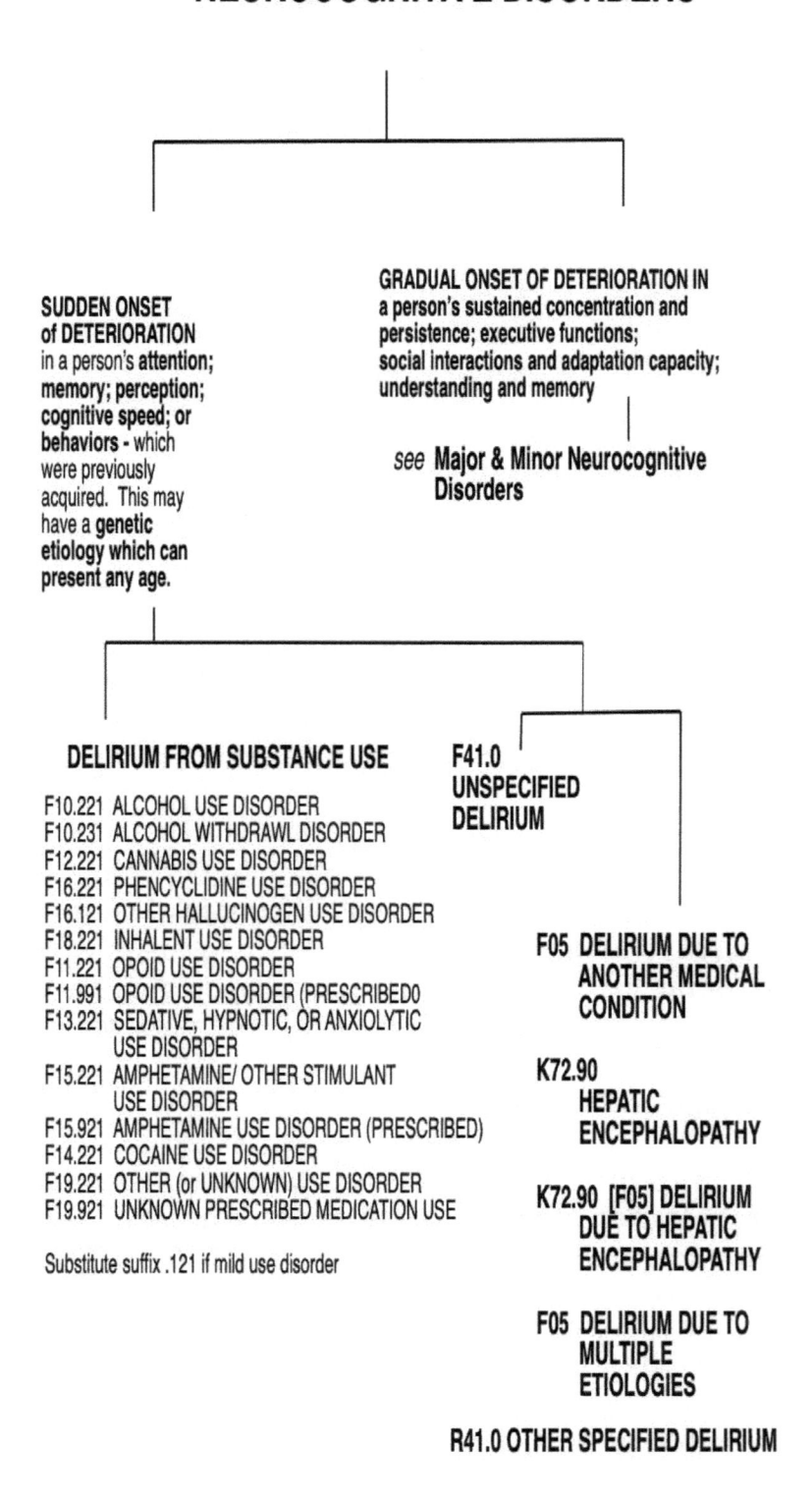

F05 DELIRIUM DUE TO ANOTHER MEDICAL CONDITION

K72.90 HEPATIC ENCEPHALOPATHY

K72.90 [F05] DELIRIUM DUE TO HEPATIC ENCEPHALOPATHY

F05 DELIRIUM DUE TO MULTIPLE ETIOLOGIES

R41.0 OTHER SPECIFIED DELIRIUM

DELIRIUM DUE TO ANOTHER MEDICAL CONDITION

ACIDOSIS (Metabolic / Respiratory)
BRAIN TUMORS / hemorrhage/ infarcts/ T.I.A.
CONVULSIONS (Partial/ Focal and Post-Ictal state)
DISORDERS OF METABOLISM
ELECTROLYTE DISORDERS
FRUCTOSE INTOLERANCE & other hypoglycemias
GLUTARIC ACIDEMIA TYPE II
HYDROCEPHALUS: increased Intracranial Pressure (ICP) & Normal-Pressure Hydrocephalus
IMMUNE DISORDERS such as AUTOIMMUNE POLYARTERITIS, INFECTIONS / ENCEPHALPATHIES of CNS
JAUNDICE & hyperammonemia & hepatic encephalopathy
KETOACIDOSIS
LACTIC ACIDOSIS
MCAD Deficiency
Neuroleptic Malignant Syndrome
Obstructive Sleep Apnea, COPD, Hypoxia/ Anoxia (Exposure to Extreme AIR PRESSURE CHANGES)
Poisons   e.g. "Glue-Sniffing" TOLUENE
Q-T Prolonged ("*Torsades de Pointes*")
Renal Tubular Acidosis
Sundowner Syndrome
Trauma (Post-Concussion Syndrome / CTE)
UREMIA / AZOTEMIA
Vitamin Deficiency (esp. B12 & Thiamine) with/without Pernicious Anemia
Wolff-Parkinson-White Syndrome with tachyarrhythmia
X-RAY (Radiation Brain necrosis after brain cancer treatment)
Yeast CNS infections
Zoster Encephalitis (HZE) & other encephalopathies

DSM-5-TR emphasizes intoxication or withdrawal from alcohol, cannabis, phencyclidine, Other hallucinogens, inhalants, opioids, sedatives-hypnotics-anxiolytics, amphetamine-type substance (or other stimulants), cocaine, and "Other (or unknown) substances". They also list "Other Specified Delirium [R41.0] and "Unspecified Delirium [R41.0].

Although the clinician is usually called to examine a patient who is in either an (1) *agitated* or (2) a *lethargic* condition, much more serious states may follow even when the pupils remain *responsive to light* including - (3) *Semi-Coma;* where there is *NO response to voice* but the patient might be aroused to *pain* (e.g., giving a "shrug" response): or (4) *Deep Metabolic Coma;* where there is *NO arousal to voice OR to pain* - where respirations are abnormal and where there may be *"gegenhalten"* or decerebrate or decorticate rigidity. A neurology consultation will usually be required in these situations. If the unfortunate patient should *show* **NO LIGHT REFLEX** of the pupils along with the above neuromuscular disorders, one should suspect (5) *Structural Brain Damage* -which is usually associated with deviation of the eyes in the resting position, with cranial nerve III, IV, and VI paresis which is detectable on the *Ice Caloric Test* or one might see the "dolls-head" response of the eyes to oculocephalic testing. Here, a Babinski reflex will often be present as will vasomotor instability. Neurosurgical consultation is required in such circumstances.

A study of the following chart, DISORDERS OF AROUSAL, can assist tracking the depth of a delirium or *Confusion State* from hyper vigilance and agitation (often present after ingesting stimulants) to *COMA* (whether following ingestion of a sedative-hypnotic-anxiolytic) or due to *Structural Brain Damage.* One score the depth of dis-arousal by utilizing the following - the **Glasgow Coma Score, Objective Neurologic Rating Scale,** or the **Objective Toxicity Rating Scale**.

DISORDERS OF AROUSAL

Impaired Attention span, Perception, Orientation for time/place/person/situation
50% loss on Immediate & Intermediate & "end of exam" Memory for 10 words

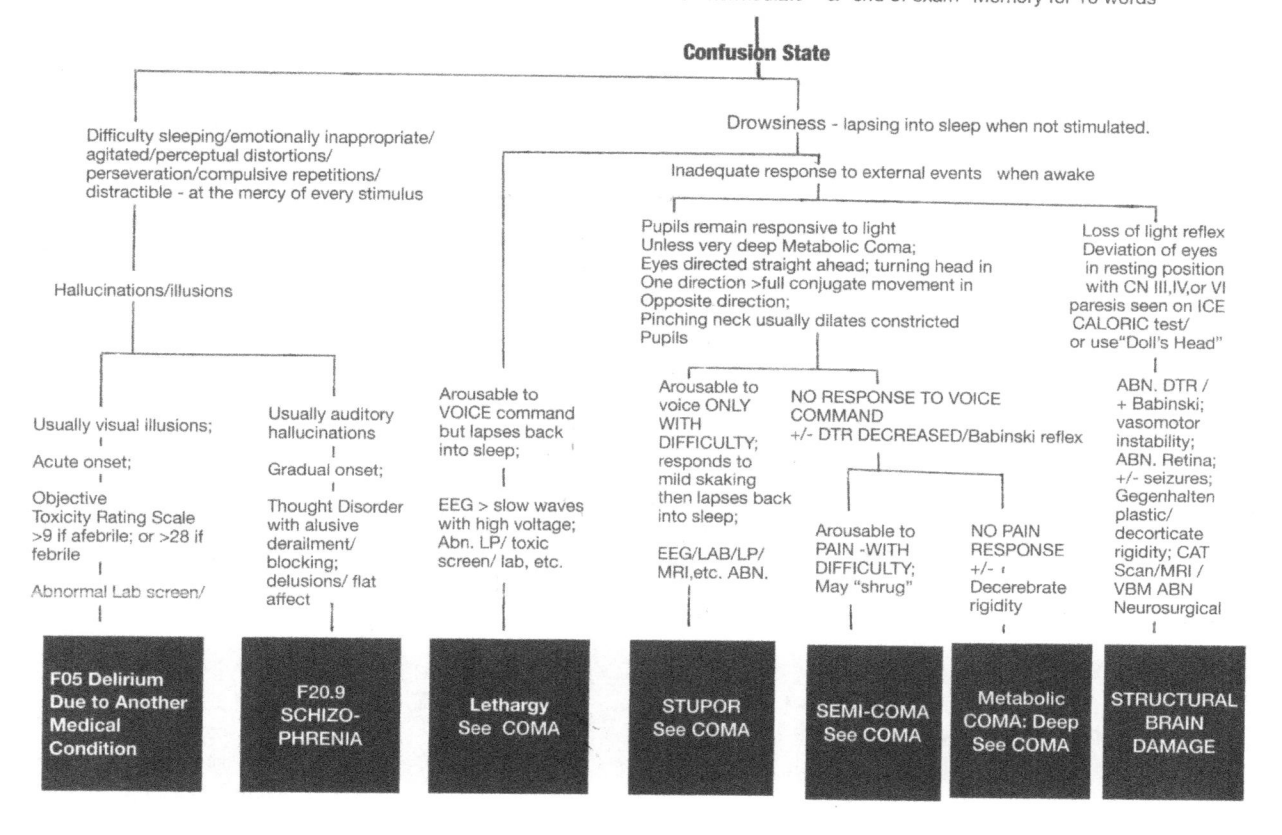

Confusion State

Branch 1: Difficulty sleeping/emotionally inappropriate/agitated/perceptual distortions/perseveration/compulsive repetitions/distractible - at the mercy of every stimulus

- Hallucinations/illusions
  - **Usually visual illusions;**
    - Acute onset;
    - Objective Toxicity Rating Scale >9 if afebrile; or >28 if febrile
    - Abnormal Lab screen/
    - → **F05 Delirium Due to Another Medical Condition**
  - **Usually auditory hallucinations**
    - Gradual onset;
    - Thought Disorder with alusive derailment/blocking; delusions/ flat affect
    - → **F20.9 SCHIZO-PHRENIA**

Branch 2: Drowsiness - lapsing into sleep when not stimulated.

Inadequate response to external events when awake

- **Arousable to VOICE command but lapses back into sleep;**
  - EEG > slow waves with high voltage; Abn. LP/ toxic screen/ lab, etc.
  - → **Lethargy See COMA**

- Pupils remain responsive to light Unless very deep Metabolic Coma; Eyes directed straight ahead; turning head in One direction >full conjugate movement in Opposite direction; Pinching neck usually dilates constricted Pupils
  - **Arousable to voice ONLY WITH DIFFICULTY; responds to mild skaking then lapses back into sleep;**
    - EEG/LAB/LP/MRI,etc. ABN.
    - → **STUPOR See COMA**
  - **NO RESPONSE TO VOICE COMMAND** +/- DTR DECREASED/Babinski reflex
    - **Arousable to PAIN -WITH DIFFICULTY; May "shrug"**
      - → **SEMI-COMA See COMA**
    - **NO PAIN RESPONSE** +/- ↑ Decerebrate rigidity
      - → **Metabolic COMA: Deep See COMA**

- Loss of light reflex Deviation of eyes in resting position with CN III,IV,or VI paresis seen on ICE CALORIC test/ or use "Doll's Head"
  - ABN. DTR / + Babinski; vasomotor instability; ABN. Retina; +/- seizures; Gegenhalten plastic/decorticate rigidity; CAT Scan/MRI / VBM ABN Neurosurgical
  - → **STRUCTURAL BRAIN DAMAGE**

TOXIC SUBSTANCES

LC = Level of Consciousness; Appear. = Appearance; ACT = Activity;

INTOXICATION SYNDROMES

Substance Class	Mental Status Exam	Physical Exam	Management
	1. LC 3.ACT. 5. Emotion 7. Orient 9. Judgment 2. Appear. 4. Speech 6.Thought Form Content 8.Memory	1. Eyes 2. B.P. 3. Pulse 4. Resp.	1. Safety 3. Antag.? 5.W/D? 2. Support 4. Symptomatic?

– –

Substance Class	Mental Status Exam	Physical Exam	Management
Sedatives/ Hypnotics	1. Obtunded 3. Disinhibited 4. Slurred 8. Poor 2. Neglected 5. Exaggerated 6. Not Goal Oriented 7. Disoriented 6. Confused/ Inappropriate 9. Poor	1. N/C 2.↓ 3.↓ 4.↓ may arrest	1. ↓stim, isolate, 2. Support 3. Antag.? 4. Symptomatic Rx ?
Opiates	1. Obtunded 4. Slurred 6. May be logical if engaged 2. Neglected 3. Disinterested 5. ↓dreamy 7. +/- 8. Poor Attention 9. Poor	1. Constricted (unless hypoxic) 2. ↓ 3. ↓ 4. ↓ may arrest	1." 2." 3. Yes: NARCAN often needs repeat doses 4. No 5. Rx w clonidine
CNS Stimulants	1. Aroused 2. Variable 3. Intrusive 4. Rapid (motor-mouth) 5. Labile/ irritable 6. LOA/ paranoia 7. +/- 8. +/- 9. Poor	1. +/- Dilated 2.↗ 3. arrhythmia 4. N/C (may seize)	1." 2." 3. NO 4. YES Haldol +cogentin or BDZ 5. NO - but may see long-lasting psychosis
Hallucinogens	1. +/- (dose-dependent); 2. +/- (occ. nudity) 3. Bizarre startling responses 4. +/-: ↓ / ↗ output 5. Excited/ scared 6. LOA/ delusions/ hallucinations 7. +/- 8. +/- 9. Poor	1. Occ. nystagmus; 2. ↓ ↗ 3. ↓ / ↗ 4.	1." 2." 3. ?Ca++ channel blockers 4. Yes " 5. No - "

GLASGOW COMA SCORE

EYE OPENING:
- 4   Spontaneous
- 3   To Speech
- 2   To Pain
- 1   None

VERBAL RESPONSE:
- 5   Oriented
- 4   Confused (may use sentences but disoriented)
- 3   Uses Inappropriate Words
- 2   Uses incomprehensible sounds
- 1   No verbal responses

BEST MOTOR RESPONSE:
- 6   Obeys commands
- 5   Localizes pain
- 4   Flexion, withdrawal to pain
- 3   Flexion - abnormal response to pain
- 2   Extension response to pain
- 1   NO response to pain

TIME: **SCORE:**   **COMMENTS:**

_____   _____   _____

_____   _____   _____

OBJECTIVE NEUROLOGIC RATING SCALE

-3	-2	-1	0	+1	+2	+3
demonstrates no ability to speak	does not understand directions &/ cannot repeat phrases	some slowness to respond	**VERBAL RESPONSES** coherent	some loose associations	very tangential; difficult to track	word salad/ verbigeration: makes no sense
shows no response	responds to only painful stimuli	responds to verbal commands	**EYE OPENING** spontaneous	fluttering while closed	staring vacantly into space	only movement is blinking eyes in response to questions
no response to light at all	constricts to not less than 5.6 mm	sluggish	**PUPILLARY REACTIONS** brisk	dilates when light moves from normal eye to this eye	responds to light but not to accommodation	pupils so constricted - can not see light reactivity
absent	roving dysconjugate	roving conjugate	**SPONTANEOUS EYE MOVEMENTS** orienting	darting	non-roving but deviation at rest position	oculogyric spasms
no response	minimal response	questionable response	**OCULOCEPHALIC RESPONSE** full conjugate eye movement opposite to direction of head turning ("dolls eyes")	patient not very cooperative	patient will not cooperate at all	head cannot be moved
no response: eyes are fixed	eyes brought to midline or slightly beyond vertical midline	eyes can be raised beyond horizontal meridian	**OCULOVESTIBULAR RESPONSE** ice caloric test shows tonic deviation to stimulated side & clonic nystagmus to opposite	patient not very cooperative	patient will not cooperate at all	test could not be performed
absent to firm touch	absent bilaterally & sensory loss scalp to light touch	questionable	**CORNEAL RESPONSE** present bilateral	absent but no loss of pain for above scalp	absent on one side	cannot be tested
apneustic: prolonged inspiratory pauses/ataxic	sustained hyperventilation	adequate ventilation: irregular patterns can't be classified	**RESPIRATORY PATTERN** regular	rapid & shallow	frequent sighing	Kussmaul deep + rapid/slow or Cheyne-Stokes

-3	-2	-1	0	+1	+2	+3
flexor spasticity or extensor rigidity	flaccid tone	Hoover's heel opposite flaccid foot exerts pressure against M.D.	**SKELETAL MUSCLE TONE** normal	"flail arm" misses face on falling	catatonic waxy flexibility	plastic rigidity
abnormal dystonic flexion or extensor spasms	appropriate movement to noxious stimuli only	responds to loud voice commands with appropriate movement	**MOTOR RESPONSE** responds to normal voice commands	does not respond to loud voice commands although awake	appropriate movement to shaking when "asleep"	no response to noxious stimuli
sustained clonus	positive Babinski reflex	+4 DTR without clonus	**DEEP TENDON REFLEXES** +2 to +3	+1 visible	+1 palpable	absent DTR

MANAGEMENT RECOMMENDATIONS:

Neurosurgical consultation ASAP for any single score of (-3) if associated with any other combination of negative scores (-3) to (-30):

Neurology consultation & toxic screen for any scores (-4) to (-13):
Neurology consultation ASAP: monitor neurological signs & vital signs & CAT scan when possible for any scores (-13)-(-33):

Psychiatric consultation for scores (+3) to (+8): & do Mental Status Exam.
Psychiatric consultation, Neurologic consultation & toxic screen laboratory testing for any score above (+8).

NOTE: to follow any condition with serial neurological ratings, disregard +/- sign and add total score for absolute value.

OBJECTIVE TOXICITY RATING SCALE

-3	-2	-1	0	+1	+2	+3
			TEMPERATURE			
96-96.7 F°	96.8-97 F°	97-97.2 F°	97.3-98.6 F°	98.7-101.9 F°	102-102.9 F°	103-104 F°
			PULSE			
45-49 adult 55-64 child	50-54 adult 65-73 child	55-61 adult 74-79 child	62-90 adult 80-110 child	91-110 adult 111-124 child	111-129 adult 125-139 child	130-149 140-150
			RESPIRATIONS			
6/min adult 8/min child	7/min adult 9-13 child	8-9 adult 14-15 child	10-16 adult 16-24 child	17-21 adult 25-29 child	22-29 adult 30-39 child	30-39 40-49
			BLOOD PRESSURE			
90/60-107/68 adult 70/48-79/49 child	108/69-110/72 adult 80/50-85/53 child	111/73-113/75 86/54-89/57	114/76-136/86 adult 90/58-106/60 child	137-87-138/88 adult 107/61-114/64 child	139/89-140/92 adult 115/65-119/67 child	above 141/93 120/68-122/72
			PUPIL SIZE			
above 7.9 mm	7.0-7.9 mm	4.0-6.9 mm	2.4-3.9 mm	2.0-2.3 mm	1.8-1.9 mm	1.6-mm or below
asleep but moves purposefully when examiner shouts	moves infrequently	sluggish	**MOTOR ACTIVITY** average movement	fidgety	hyperactive	wild thrashing
asleep but wakens easily to shouting	sleepy but attends to loud voice	attends with effort	**AROUSAL STATE** alert	attends but distracted	short attention span	distracted by every stimulus
flat affect & uninterested	somewhat flat & withdrawn	quiet but will converse/play	**MOOD** friendly/playful	serious but will engage in conversation/play	fussy & doesn't want to interact	very irritable & uncooperative
cannot be consoled	can be consoled with much effort	can be consoled with some effort	**CONSOLABILITY** average	distracted easily from distress	doesn't focus on illness/pain	seems unaware of the illness/pain
ashen gray	very pale	some pallor	**COLOR** unremarkable	flushed face	red face	beet red
cold & clammy skin or swollen around eyes/2+ edema	1+ ankle edema	± ankle edema	**HYDRATION** unremarkable	decreased tears	dry mucous membranes	dry skin; sunken eyes; tenting or doughy skin

SCORING: add all numbers - disregard +/- sign to get absolute value: if absolute value above 11 do CBC, ESR; above 19 do CXR & SMAC$_{20}$; TSH do toxic screen EKG, T$_4$ & T$_3$, UA & monitor I & O: follow-up with Objective Neurological Rating Scale.
Scoring should be performed when patient is in optimal state: after 20 minutes rest & antipyretic medication administration

NeuroCognitive Disorder Due to Another Medical Condition

OFTEN SUDDEN ONSET OF CONFUSION/ DISORIENTATION/ LETHARGY/STUPOR/IRRITABILITY
+/- headache/ dizziness/vertigo/ataxia or clumsy gait or stance/blurred vision/ seizures
+/- nausea/ vomiting/ history of ingestion/ inhalation of toxic materials

NO EVIDENCE OF STRUCTURAL COMA SIGNS ON NEUROLOGICAL & CT EXAMS

METABOLIC STUPOR/COMA DUE TO POISONS

PALLOR/ CYANOSIS

SKIN MAY BE CHERRY RED
+/- glycosuria; signs of INC. Intracranial Pressure;

IMPROVES with 20-40 Oxygen RX/

Dexamethasone for CNS edema

CARBON MONOXIDE POISONING/ SMOKE INHALATION

STIFF LOWER JAW; BREATH IS ODOR OF BITTER ALMONDS
Hyperpnea/ prolonged respirations

Follows **ingestion** of silver polish/ photo chems/ elderberry leaves/ cherry/ peach/ apricot pits/

CYANIDE POISONING

TACHYPNEA
follows ingestion of WELL water

diarrhea/ diuresis;

oximetry suggests methemo-globinemia

Rx with O2 & methylene blue

NITRITE/ NITRATE POISONING

+/- LEG MUSCLE CRAMPS/ VASO-MOTOR DISTURBANCES;
Inc. Serum Amylase PANCREATITIS

HX ingestion Paint removers/ varnish/ STERNO/ anti-freeze/ wood alcohol

Rx with ETHANOL 1-2 oz./ hour Bicarb & hemo- or peritoneal dialysis

METHANOL TOXICITY (Wood Alcohol)

MUSCLE PARALYSIS
RHODODENDRON POISONING

diarrhea/ gangrene of digits after migraine RX **ingestion** of ergotamine

ERGOT POISONING

CRAMPING/ ABDOMINAL PAIN

DIARRHEA/ RENAL DAMAGE
R/O NAPHTHALENE/ LEAD/ YELLOW PHOSPHOROUS or ARSENIC POISONING

CHLORINATED HYDROCARBON TOXICITY

DELIRIUM: DIFFERENTIAL DIAGNOSIS

Instructions: Place an "X" in appropriate box if the problem is present.

PROBLEM	DIAGNOSIS
Generalized convulsions	Occasional seizures / Status Epilepticus
Headache, vomiting, dizziness, blurred vision, shock, R.D.S.	Cerebral Edema
History/ PE of Head Injury: skull films normal	Mild Head Injury
Loss of consciousness less than 1 hr: persistent but non-progressive neuro Sx	Moderate Head Injury
Loss of consciousness greater than 1 hr; abnormal neuro signs develop and persist but there is no deterioration:	Severe Head Injury
or neuro status deteriorates ± decorticate/decerebrate ± skull fracture	Epidural/subdural Hematoma
Nuchal rigidity ± sensory losses & quadriparesis	Cervical Spine Fracture
Constricted pupils	
Pupils don't dilate on neck-pinching: ± conjugate deviation of eyes at rest: ± lesion CN VI/VII & UMN lesion X,XI,XII ± central neurogenic hyperventilation.	Pontine structural lesion
Pupils may dilate on neck-pinching/light reflex may be present	
History of ingestion of toxins or gas/drugs	
Abdominal cramps ± diarrhea ± wheezing	
Tachycardia/hypertension/nystagmus	PCP Toxicity
Bradycardia/dropped beats c̄ block; muscle twitches or fasciculations then paralysis & loss sphincter control	
Liver/renal damage: Hx eating mushrooms	Mushroom Poisoning
Hx contact with insecticide (e.g. Malathion)	Organic Phosphate Poisoning
Respiration depressed ± pulmonary edema: scars, needle tracts ± phlebitis: follows use of opiates/ narcotics/propoxyphene (occ. phenothiazine/sedative)	Narcotic Poisoning

COMA: SUDDEN ONSET AFTER TOXIC EXPOSURE — DIAGNOSIS

CONVULSIONS: generalized± cerabral hypoxia; may be preceded by headache, dizziness, vertigo, ataxia, blurred vision, ± R.D.S. ± shock

DILATED PUPILS

GASTROENTERITIS ± abdominal pain ± diarrhea	
Follows ingestion of ergotamine/ Sansert: ± pancreatitis, muscle cramps, hypocalcemia, cold gangrenous extremities	Ergot Poisoning
RENAL DAMAGE ± proteinuria, oliguria or shutdown	
Hemolytic anemia ± hemoglobinuria after ingestion of mothballs or deodorant cakes	Naphthalene Poisoning
X-RAY MAY SHOW RADIOOPACITY OF HEAVY METAL	
Hemolysis ± pulmonary edema: increased DTR	Arsenic
Hemolytic anemia & hemoglobinemia after ingestion of lead-paint/ inhaling gasoline or burning newspaper logs: urine porphyrins inc.	Lead Poisoning
Hepatic necrosis after rodenticide ingestion or mercury amalgam	Inorganic Mercury
Hepatic necrosis/ shock/ melena/ coagulation defects after ingesting iron (ferrous/ferric sulfate)	Iron Poisoning
Hepatic necrosis ± jaundice, hypoglycemia, hemorrhage into skin or mucosa: garlic odor to breath: may follow several days after ingestion of insecticides or fireworks: ± skin burns	Yellow Phosphorous Poisoning

___HYPERVENTILATION

   ___RESPIRATORY ALKALOSIS

      ___Purpura, hematemesis, tachycardia ± fever   D.I.C.

      ___Jaundice, abnormally large/shrunken liver with abnormal liver battery   HEPATIC ENCEPHALOPATHY

      ___Cyanosis, heart murmur ± rales in cardiopulmonary disease   CHF --CONGENITAL HEART DISEASE

      ___Absent pupillary & vestibular responses ± CN disorders in CNS disorder   NEUROGENIC HYPERVENTILATION

___HYPOVENTILATION ± CYANOSIS & RESPIRATORY ACIDOSIS

   ___NEUROMUSCULAR WEAKNESS

      ___Descending weakness ± ptosis, nystagmus, dry throat, inability to support head, dysphagia, dysphonia

         ___Pharyngeal pain, nausea, vomiting p eating home-canned alkaline foods   BOTULISM

         ___Responds to 0.2 mg/kg (adult max= 5 mg) Tensilon   MYASTHENIA GRAVIS

         ___Fascicluations with increased DTR   FAMILIAL ALS (WERD. HOFFMAN, ET

         ___Hypoglycemia with Hx chronic hypoglycemia   CHRONIC HYPOCLYCEMIA

      ___Ascending weakness ± paresthesiae, dec. touch, pain & vibration

         ___Follows barbiturate/sulfonamides; + urine Watson-Schwartz   ACUTE INTERMITTENT PORPHYRIA

         ___Macrocytosis & B_{12} or folate deficiency   SUBACUTE COMBINED DEGENERATION

         ___Fever, multiple systemic involvement, + FANA & inc. ESR   AUTO-IMMUNE ARTERITIS

         ___After chronic exposure to toxins (heavy metals, ortho cresyl phosphate)   TOXIC NEUROPATHY

         ___After chronic diabetes and hyperglycemia   DIABETIC NEUROPATHY

   ___CHEST TRAUMA after auto accident, severe kyphoscoliosis, flail chest   CHEST COMPRESSION

   ___OBESITY with compromised ventilation   PICKWICK'S SYNDROME

___HYPOVENTILATION ± CYANOSIS & METABOLIC ALKALOSIS

    ___Truncal obesity, hirsutism, hypertension, bruises, purple striae   CUSHING'S SYNDROME

    ___History of hypertension treated with diuretics   DRUG ALKALOSIS

    ___Hypertension ± periodic paralysis, inc. plasma Na^+, polyuria   HYPERALDOSTERONSIM

    ___Hypokalemia, urine Cl^- wasting with hypochloremia (inc. aldosterone & renin)   BARTTER'S SYNDROME

___HYPERTENSION

    ___Diastolic BP greater than 120, retinal artery spasms ± hemorrhage; EKG LVH/strain   HYPERTENSIVE ENCEPHALOPATHY

    ___Nausea, vomiting, diarrhea, autonomic storm ± "dancing eyes-dancing feet"   PHEO/ NEURAL CREST TUMOR

    ___Goiter, tremor, heat intolerance, fine hair, autonomic storm as above   HYPERTHYROIDISM

___HYPOTENSION

    ___Greater than 20 point deficit in BP on standing   POSTURAL HYPOTENSION

    ___Carotid sinus pressure causes fainting
        ___Adolescent; BP drop corrected by 0.5 cc epinephrine (1:1000)   VASOMOTOR/VASODEPRESSOR SYNCOPE
        ___Older pt. with bradycardia corrected by 1 mg Atropine   VAGAL TYPE CAROTID SINUS SYNCOPE

___BRADYCARDIA: PULSE LESS THAN 60 IN CHILDREN

    ___Sinus bradycardia; non-phasic with respiration: ± SA block/ paroxysmal arrhythmia   SICK SINUS SYNDROME/MYOCARDIOPATH

    ___EKG p waves have no relation to QRS complex 3° HEART BLOCK

    ___Dropped beats not preceded by progressive delay of previous P-R interval but Atropine challenge reveals concealed heart block 2^O BLOCK: MOBITZ TYPE II

    Stokes-Adams Syndrome

___TACHYCARDIA

    Reg. rhythm & R-R interval, each p followed by normal QRS   SUPRAVENTRICULAR TACHYCARDIA

___FEVER
    ___Purpura, hypotension, shock   D.I.C.

    ___Meningismus, abnormal CSF WBC's /glucose   CNS INFECTION

    ___Meningismus, CSF increased RBC   S.A.H. **SubArachnoid Hemorrhage**

___MYXEDEMA, goiter, coarse hair, thick tongue, bradycardia, "water bottle heart" on CXR   HYPOTHYROIDISM

___MUSCLE SPASMS: trismus, + Chvostek sign/carpopedal spasm   HYPOCALCEMIA/HYPOMAGNESEMIA

___HYPONATREMIA (110-120);hypoosmolal serum & inappropriate concentrated urine   INAPPROPRIATE ADH SYNDROME
                                        & dilute urine   DIETARY DISORDER INFANCY
___HYPERNATREMIA (above 155) or HYPOPROTEINEMIA on SPE or POLYCYTHEMIA (above 65-70)   HYPERVISCOSITY SYNDROME

___HYPOGLYCEMIA ± diabetic on insulin: moist, pale skin, shallow respiration; inc. DTR   HYPOGLYCEMIA

___NORMAL PHYSICAL EXAM   MANIC AFFECTIVE DISORDER

Assistance from pediatric or metabolic consultation will be required on most of the above disorders with the exception of uncomplicated chronic diarrhea, diabetes mellitus, acute intermittent porphyria, COPD, syncope, meningitis or viral encephalitis.

This chapter will attempt to give the clinician a methodical approach to the symptoms presented by patients presenting in a **confusion state** of DELIRIUM. (Of course mixed pictures will present in such illnesses as Multiple Sclerosis and Systemic Lupus Erythematosis). Since all causes of Delirium must first be assumed to have an organic etiology, the discussion will include the Neurocognitive Disorders Due to Another Medical Condition.

Delirium may be defined as a confusion state with an onset of symptoms in hours or days, and with symptoms which usually flucuate over time. There must be two cognitive impairments:

1. Recent onset of an Attention Deficit: e.g.

    a. Test for Auditory Attention scores <70 % expected for age;(see p. 80)

    b. Speech may be repetitive or perseverative;

    c. For an adult, Digit Span is < 5 numbers (forward) and < 4 numbers backward.

    d. Or Psychological Testing with the Stroop Test shows > 30% failed responses.

    e. Concentration or Processing Speed will show mistakes or problems on the Serial-7 subtraction test (adults) or Serial-3 subtraction Test (on younger children) - or else the examiner will not an abnormal speed of response to the examiner's questions. This may be elicited in one of 4 ways:

    (1). Patient takes abnormally long time to respond to questions;

    (2). Patient shows extreme distractibility and is "at the mercy of every stimulus): "impersistence" in general or evidenced by specific questioning. Or,

    (3). Patient gives rapid or "flippant" responses, speaking rapidly; Or

f. Failure to carry out simple commands: e.g.,

(1) ONE-STEP COMMAND: "Take this pencil with your left hand";

(2) TWO-STEP COMMAND: "Use the pencil to write your complete name"; and

(3) THREE-STEP COMMAND: "Give me back the pencil using your right hand".

A child at age 5 should be able to complete a 3-Stage Command without difficulty. Instead of asking a child to "Write your complete name" the examiner could ask: "Fold this paper in half" - using paper instead of "Take this pencil".

2. There is an ADDITIONAL COGNITIVE DEFICIT ALSO OF RECENT ONSET: this may manifest in deficits of:

a. **ORIENTATION:** with confusion about:

(1) Todays DATE / month / year;

(2) Current PLACE: "Where are you now?"; or

(3) CIRCUMSTANCE: "Why are you here?": or

b. **PERCEPTUAL ERRORS** - when asked to:

(1) "Draw the Face of a clock showing 5 minutes past 11 o'clock"; or

(2) Failing the Bender Test of designs; or Beery-Buktenica standardized designs; or the "Draw-A-Person" which may show missing parts of a body or only a "stick-figure".

(3) Show "Popular Pull": e.g. on the Roberts-2 Cognitive Test; or

(4) Grasp the **meaning** of proverbs or questions asked the patient.

Since DSM-5 Diagnosis of DELIRIUM requires CATEGORY E: History, Physical, Laboratory or X-Ray studies support medical causes such as substance intoxication or withdrawn; toxic chemical etiology; or medication adverse effects - LABORATORY STUDIES including a Toxic Drug Screen and CAT scan of the brain should be ordered - as well as blood levels of expected medications.

The following **checklist** might aid in the diagnosis of **"DELIRIUM DUE TO ANOTHER MEDICAL CONDITION"**:

LABORATORY INVESTIGATION FOR NEUROLOGICAL DISORDER DUE TO ANOTHER MEDICAL CONDITION

ICD-10-CM	DIAGNOSIS: DELIRIUM DUE TO -	TESTS:
E 87.2 (F05)	**ACIDOSIS: METABOLIC**	BLOOD GASES: STAT; ON ICE; LACTATE & PYRUVATE & SERUM ELECTROLYTES;BUN
E 27.40 (F05)	- ADRENAL INSUFFICIENCY	SERUM CORTISOL,; ACTH;
E 05.11 (F05)	- THYROTOXICOSIS; GRAVE'S DISEASE	RAI131 UPTAKE; TSH; T4;T3; thyroglobulin; antimicrosomal & thyroid auto-ab & scan
E 87.2 (F05)	- LACTIC ACIDOSIS	Urine pH & Ketones; Benedict Test for Reducing Substances- if +,do Chromatography
R 40.20 (F05)	- DIABETIC/ ANOXIC LACTIC ACIDOSIS	TO DISCERN WHICH SUGAR IS PRESENT; SAMPLE AMINO & ORGANIC ACIDS; TRIGLYCERID
	- DISORDER OF FATTY ACID OXIDATION MCAD DEFICIENCY;	Cholesterol; uric acid; transaminases; creatinine & carnitine; homocystine;profile acyl carnitine esters; inc. octanoyl carnitine & dec. excretion of ketones in presence of hexanoyl glycine when client is ill ; CPK Kinase(CK)
E 08.11/10(F05)	DIABETIC ketoacidosis w/wo COMA	INCREASED URINE KETONES X 2
	DISORDERS OF ENERGY METABOLISM/ CARBOHYDRATE METABOLISM/ ORGANIC ACID METABOLISM/PURINE METABOLISM/ PEROXISOMES/LYSOSOMAL STORAGE DISEASE/ STARVATION/KETOSIS/CHRONIC DIARRHEA/GLUTARIC ACIDEMIA TYPE II/ ALDOSTERONE DEFICIT/UNRESPON.	
	ACIDOSIS: RESPIRATORY	
	- **ACUTE INTERMITTENT PORPHYRIA**	PORPHOBILINOGENS; URINE; AMINOLEVULINIC ACID; Porphobilinogen synthase level (delta amino levuliic acid dehydrogenase) ALAD GENE
	- **COPD**	CHEST X-RAY; pA02; oximetry
	- AUTOIMMUNE POLYARTERITIS	
	- MYASTHENIA GRAVIS	TENSILON TEST 0.2 MG/KG (MA 5 MG ADULTS)
	- BOTULISM	
	ALKALOSIS: RESPIRATORY	Nuclear stress test/MUGA or ECHOCARDIOGRAM/MRI SCAN OF
Q 24.9 (F05)	- CONGENITAL HEART DISEASE:FAILURE	HEART > ejection fraction <40% HF-rEF/pEF;
	- HEPATIC ENCEPHALOPATHY	Free-Flowing Blood AMMONIA; LIVER FUNCTION TESTS including clotting tests to confirm liver failure; platelets <100;
	— DISSEMINATED INTRAVASCULAR COAG	+Fibrin Degradation Products; inc. Prothrombin time; Fibrinogen <1
	ALKALOSIS: METABOLIC	BLOOD GASES: STAT; ON ICE;
E 34.9 (F05)	- CUSHING'S SYNDROME	Overnight low-dose DEXAMETASONE SUPPRESSION TEST
R 40.20 (F05)	- DIURETIC ALKALOSIS	BLOOD GASES: STAT; ON ICE; BP HX; MED HX

LABORATORY INVESTIGATION FOR NEUROCOGNITIVE DISORDER DUE TO ANOTHER MEDICAL CONDITION

ICD-10-CM	DIAGNOSIS: DELIRIUM DUE TO -	TESTS
	BRAIN TUMORS	MRI WITH CONTRAST; CT SCAN HEAD
	CIRCULATORY	CARDIAC ULTRASONOGRAPHY; CAROTID DOPPLER
R 40.20 (F05)	- HYPERTENSION ENCEPHALOPATHY	BP DIASTOLIC >120; SYSTOLIC >180
	- PHEOCHROMOCYTOMA	Urine Metanephrines; Blood catecholamines or 24 hr urine; MIB6 Scintigraphy 123 or PET-MRI
I 95 (F05)	- HYPOTENSION	BP MONITORING; VITAL SIGNS, ETC.
I 65.29 (F05)	- CAROTID STENOSIS	CEREBRAL ANGIOGRAPHY; CAROTID DUPLEX; MAGNETIC RESONANCE ANGIOGRAPHY (MRA)
R00.1 (F05)	BRADYCARDIA, UNSPECIFIED	ECG; KING OF HEARTS STUDY X 1 MO; HOLTER MONITOR
I 49.5 (F05)	- SICK SINUS SYNDROME	ECG; KING OF HEARTS STUDY X 1 MO; HOLTER MONITOR
F07.81 (F05)	**CONCUSSION: POST-CONCUSSION SYNDROME**	NON-CONTRAST HEAD CT
S 06.0	-CNS TRAUMA	
S 06.4 (F05)	-DELIRIUM DUE TO EPIDURAL HEMORRHAGE	SERIAL HEAD CT SHOWS LENS-SHAPED HYPER-DENSITY/ MRI
I 62.01 (F05)	- DELIRIUM DUE TO SUBDURAL HEMATOMA	CT HEAD & SPINE SHOWS CLASSIC "CRESCENT BETWEEN BRAIN & INNER TABLE OF SKULL)
	CEREBRAL TUMOR	MRI HEAD WITH CONTRAST
	CONVULSIONS	ABNORMAL EEG DURING SEIZURE
G 40.0 (F05)	- LOCALIZED/FOCAL/PARTIAL SEIZURES	MAY SEE TEMPORAL LOBE SPIKES 2 WKS AFTER SEIZURE
	ELECTROLYTE DISORDERS	
E 22.2 (F05)	- SYNDROME OF INAPPROPRIATE ADH SECRETION	EXTRACELLULAR OSMOLALITY <270 mOsm;/kg; urine concentration >100 mOsm/kg; no hx diuretic use

LABORATORY INVESTIGATION FOR NEUROLOGICAL DISORDER DUE TO ANOTHER MEDICAL CONDITION

ICD-10-CM	DIAGNOSIS	TESTS
	CEREBRAL HEMORRHAGE	
I 62.01 (F05)	- SUBDURAL HEMATOMA	CT HEAD & SPINE (Classic "crescent" between brain & inner table of skull
S 06.4x9A (F05)	- EPIDURAL HEMATOMA	
	CEREBRAL ISCHEMIA	
G45.9 (F05)	STENOSIS CAROTID ARTERY;T.I.A.; Atherosclerosis	CAROTID DOPPLER - ULTRASONOGRAPHY
Z86.73 (F05)	STENOSIS VERTEBRO-BASILAR ARTERY T.I.A.	TRANSCRANIAL DOPPLER ULTRASONOGRAPHY
I77.3 (F05)	Carotid Artery FIBROMUSCULAR DYSPLASIA	MRI CEREBRAL ARTERIOGRAPHY
I 48.1 (F05)	CAROTID THROMBUS - ATRIAL FIBRILLATION	EKG; CAROTID DOPPLER
G 31.9 (F05)	CNS LACULAR STATE	MRI BRAIN
I 34.2 (F05)	MITRAL STENOSIS	CARDIAC SONOGRAPHY (ECHOCARDIOGRAM)
D 57.21 (F05)	SICKLE-CELL EMBOLIC PROCESS	SICKLE PREP
I 27.9 (F05)	PULMONARY HYPOPERFUSION	CHEST X-RAY; OXIMETRY
F 07.81 (F05)	**CEREBRAL TRAUMA (TRI/ CTE)**	NON-CONTRAST HEAD CT SCAN
	HYDROCEPHALUS (INC.NORM. PRESSURE)	CT SCAN HEAD; NEUROLOGY (LP)
F 32.15 (F05)	**IMMUNE DISORDERS**	ANTI-SSA;ANTI-SSB; ANTI-RNP ANTIBODIES; RPR; ESR;
	SYSTEMIC LUPUS ERYTHEMATOSIS	L.E. PREP FANA;ANTICOAGULANT ANTI-DNA; ANTI-HISTONE/ SMITH
M 30 (F05)	AUTOIMMUNE POLYARTERITIS SJOGREN	
A81	**INFECTIOUS DISORDERS**	CBC; BLOOD CULTURES/ VIRAL STUDIES
A85	ENCEPHALITIS	LP; SPECIFIC CULTURES MRI
A 52.1 (F05)	SYSTEMIC NEUROSYPHILIS	VDRL; FTA-ABS; (FLUORESCENT TREPONEMA ANTIBODY ABSORBED)
G 47.33 (F05)	**OBSTRUCTIVE SLEEP APNEA**	SLEEP STUDIES - POLYSOMNOGRAPHY

DELIRIUM with Headache +/- Neurological Signs

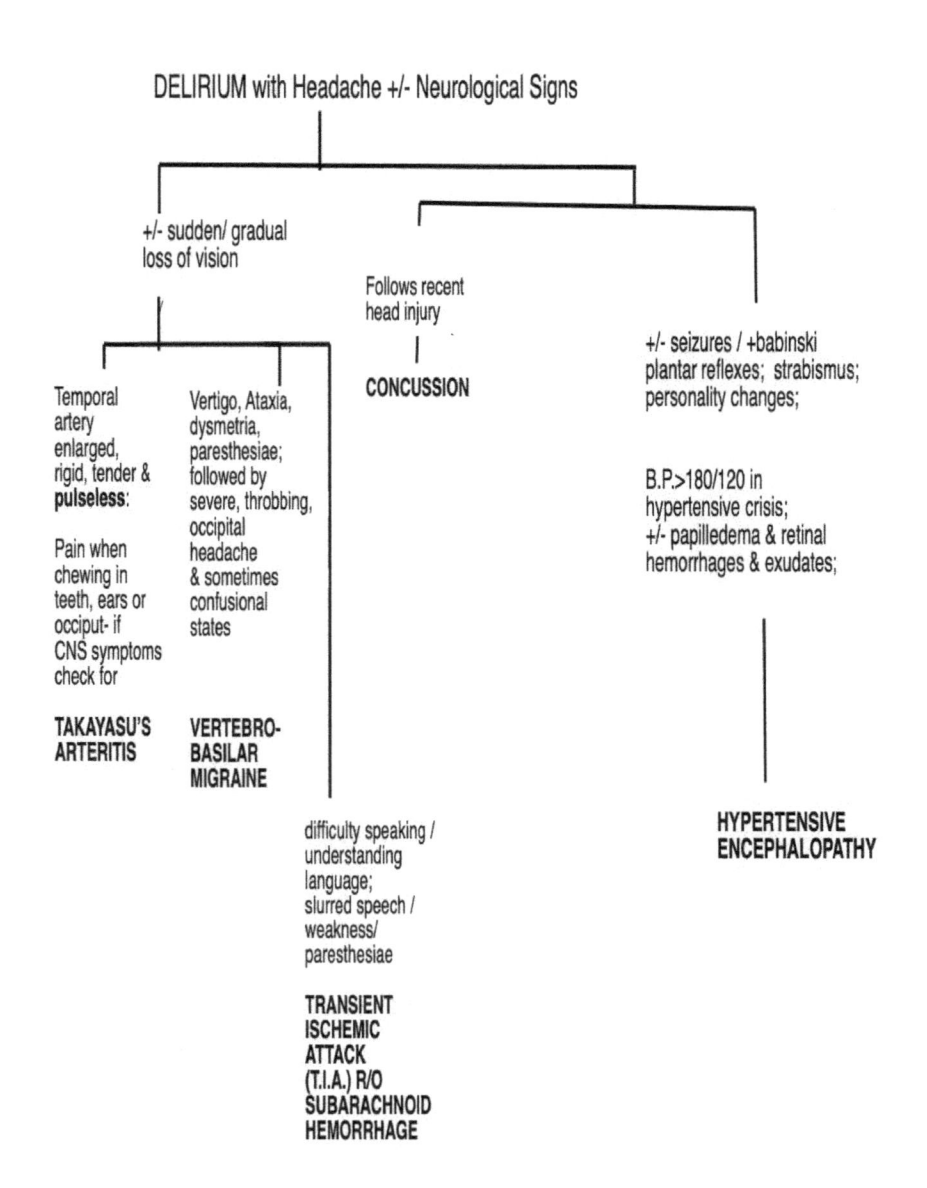

+/- sudden/ gradual loss of vision

Temporal artery enlarged, rigid, tender & **pulseless**:
Pain when chewing in teeth, ears or occiput- if CNS symptoms check for

TAKAYASU'S ARTERITIS

Vertigo, Ataxia, dysmetria, paresthesiae; followed by severe, throbbing, occipital headache & sometimes confusional states

VERTEBRO-BASILAR MIGRAINE

difficulty speaking / understanding language; slurred speech / weakness/ paresthesiae

TRANSIENT ISCHEMIC ATTACK (T.I.A.) R/O SUBARACHNOID HEMORRHAGE

Follows recent head injury

CONCUSSION

+/- seizures / +babinski plantar reflexes; strabismus; personality changes;

B.P.>180/120 in hypertensive crisis; +/- papilledema & retinal hemorrhages & exudates;

HYPERTENSIVE ENCEPHALOPATHY

DELIRIUM DUE TO HYPERCALCEMIA

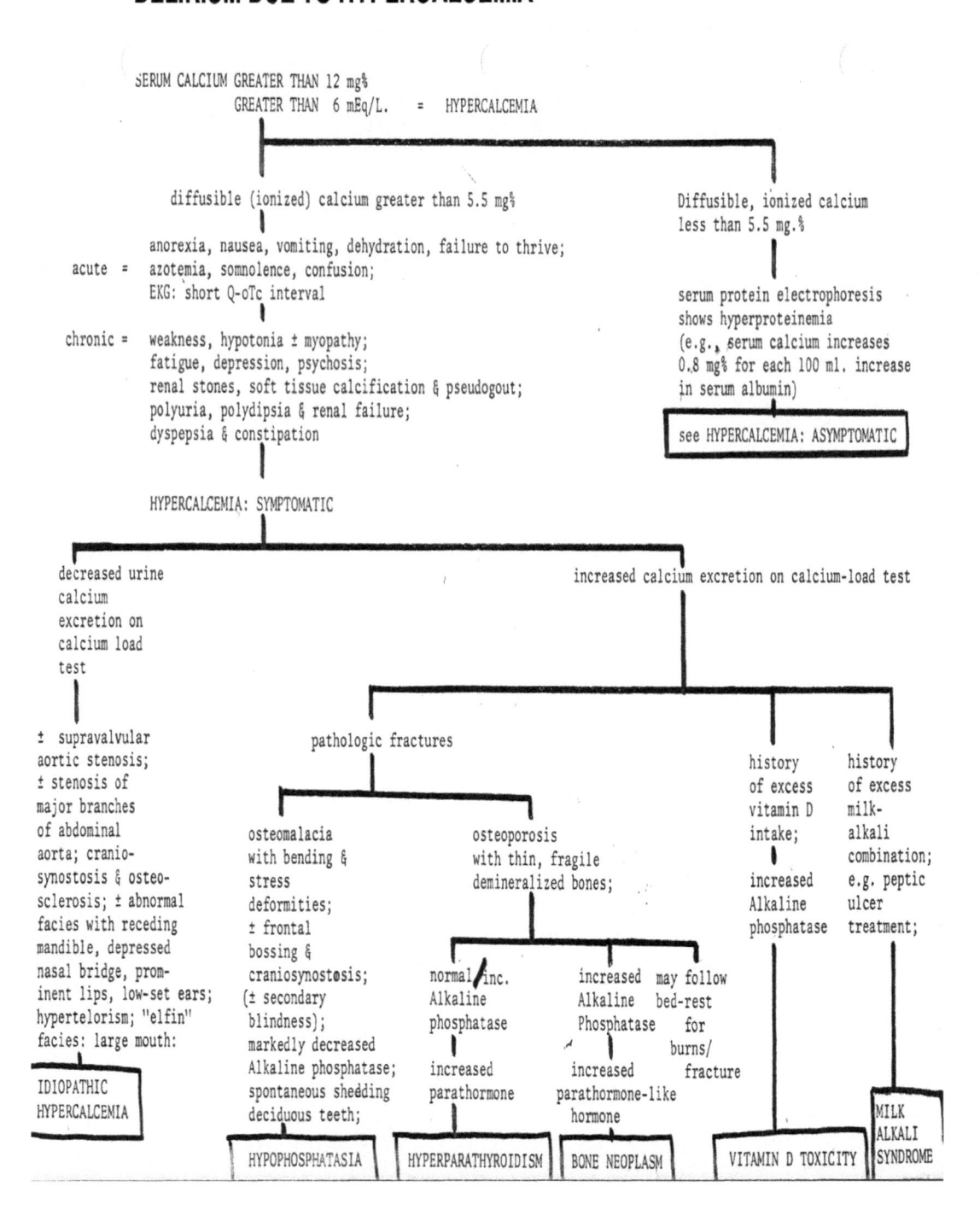

SERUM CALCIUM GREATER THAN 12 mg%
            GREATER THAN 6 mEq/L.   =   HYPERCALCEMIA

diffusible (ionized) calcium greater than 5.5 mg%

acute =
- anorexia, nausea, vomiting, dehydration, failure to thrive;
- azotemia, somnolence, confusion;
- EKG: short Q-oTc interval

chronic =
- weakness, hypotonia ± myopathy;
- fatigue, depression, psychosis;
- renal stones, soft tissue calcification & pseudogout;
- polyuria, polydipsia & renal failure;
- dyspepsia & constipation

Diffusible, ionized calcium less than 5.5 mg.%

serum protein electrophoresis shows hyperproteinemia (e.g., serum calcium increases 0.8 mg% for each 100 ml. increase in serum albumin)

see HYPERCALCEMIA: ASYMPTOMATIC

HYPERCALCEMIA: SYMPTOMATIC

decreased urine calcium excretion on calcium load test

increased calcium excretion on calcium-load test

± supravalvular aortic stenosis; ± stenosis of major branches of abdominal aorta; craniosynostosis & osteosclerosis; ± abnormal facies with receding mandible, depressed nasal bridge, prominent lips, low-set ears; hypertelorism; "elfin" facies: large mouth:

IDIOPATHIC HYPERCALCEMIA

pathologic fractures

osteomalacia with bending & stress deformities; ± frontal bossing & craniosynostosis; (± secondary blindness); markedly decreased Alkaline phosphatase; spontaneous shedding deciduous teeth;

HYPOPHOSPHATASIA

osteoporosis with thin, fragile demineralized bones;

normal/inc. Alkaline phosphatase

increased parathormone

HYPERPARATHYROIDISM

increased Alkaline Phosphatase

increased parathormone-like hormone

BONE NEOPLASM

may follow bed-rest for burns/ fracture

history of excess vitamin D intake;

increased Alkaline phosphatase

VITAMIN D TOXICITY

history of excess milk-alkali combination; e.g. peptic ulcer treatment;

MILK ALKALI SYNDROME

DELIRIUM DUE TO ANOTHER MEDICATION CONDITION

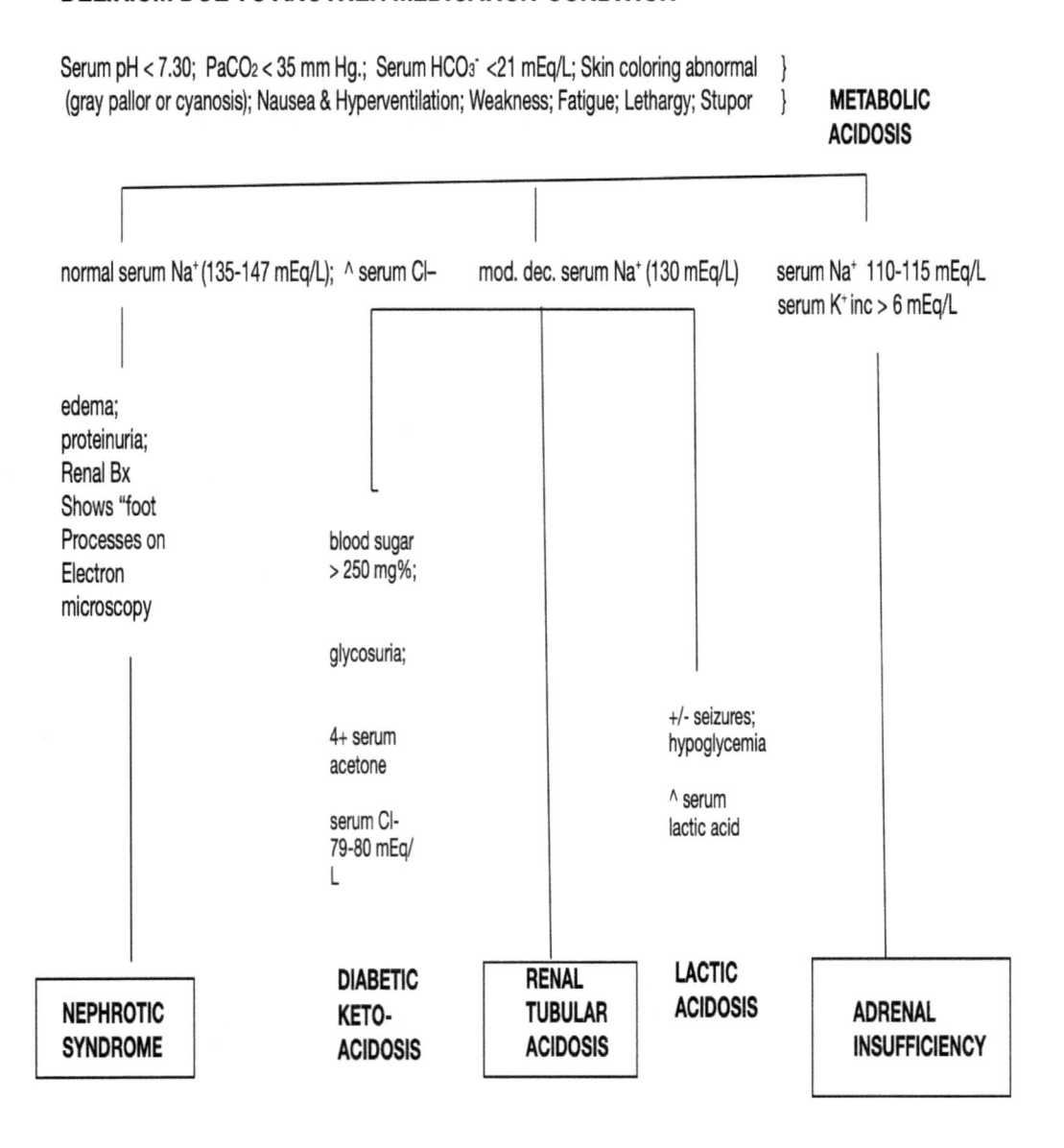

Serum pH < 7.30; PaCO$_2$ < 35 mm Hg.; Serum HCO$_3^-$ <21 mEq/L; Skin coloring abnormal } **METABOLIC**
(gray pallor or cyanosis); Nausea & Hyperventilation; Weakness; Fatigue; Lethargy; Stupor } **ACIDOSIS**

normal serum Na$^+$ (135-147 mEq/L); ^ serum Cl– | mod. dec. serum Na$^+$ (130 mEq/L) | serum Na$^+$ 110-115 mEq/L; serum K$^+$ inc > 6 mEq/L

- edema; proteinuria; Renal Bx Shows "foot Processes on Electron microscopy

- blood sugar > 250 mg%;
- glycosuria;
- 4+ serum acetone
- serum Cl- 79-80 mEq/L

- +/- seizures; hypoglycemia
- ^ serum lactic acid

| NEPHROTIC SYNDROME | DIABETIC KETO-ACIDOSIS | RENAL TUBULAR ACIDOSIS | LACTIC ACIDOSIS | ADRENAL INSUFFICIENCY |

DELIRIUM DUE TO ANOTHER MEDICAL CONDITION

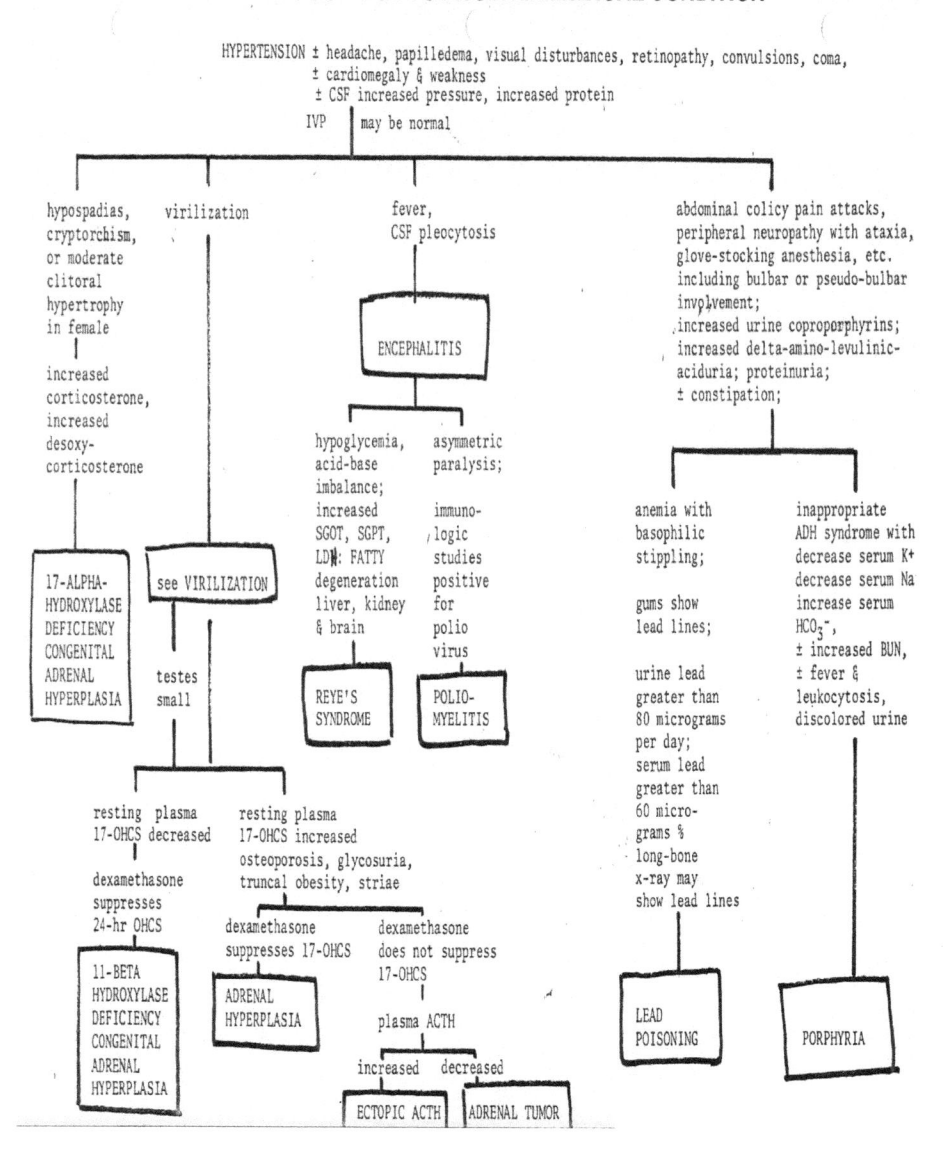

HYPERTENSION ± headache, papilledema, visual disturbances, retinopathy, convulsions, coma,
± cardiomegaly & weakness
± CSF increased pressure, increased protein
IVP may be normal

hypospadias, cryptorchism, or moderate clitoral hypertrophy in female

increased corticosterone, increased desoxy-corticosterone

17-ALPHA-HYDROXYLASE DEFICIENCY CONGENITAL ADRENAL HYPERPLASIA

virilization

see VIRILIZATION

testes small

resting plasma 17-OHCS decreased

dexamethasone suppresses 24-hr OHCS

11-BETA HYDROXYLASE DEFICIENCY CONGENITAL ADRENAL HYPERPLASIA

resting plasma 17-OHCS increased
osteoporosis, glycosuria, truncal obesity, striae

dexamethasone suppresses 17-OHCS

ADRENAL HYPERPLASIA

dexamethasone does not suppress 17-OHCS

plasma ACTH

- increased → **ECTOPIC ACTH**
- decreased → **ADRENAL TUMOR**

fever, CSF pleocytosis

ENCEPHALITIS

hypoglycemia, acid-base imbalance; increased SGOT, SGPT, LDH: FATTY degeneration liver, kidney & brain

REYE'S SYNDROME

asymmetric paralysis; immunologic studies positive for polio virus

POLIOMYELITIS

abdominal colicky pain attacks, peripheral neuropathy with ataxia, glove-stocking anesthesia, etc. including bulbar or pseudo-bulbar involvement;
increased urine coproporphyrins;
increased delta-amino-levulinic-aciduria; proteinuria;
± constipation;

anemia with basophilic stippling;
gums show lead lines;
urine lead greater than 80 micrograms per day;
serum lead greater than 60 micrograms %
long-bone x-ray may show lead lines

LEAD POISONING

inappropriate ADH syndrome with decrease serum K+ decrease serum Na increase serum HCO_3^-,
± increased BUN,
± fever & leukocytosis,
discolored urine

PORPHYRIA

DELIRIUM DUE TO ANOTHER MEDICAL CONDITION

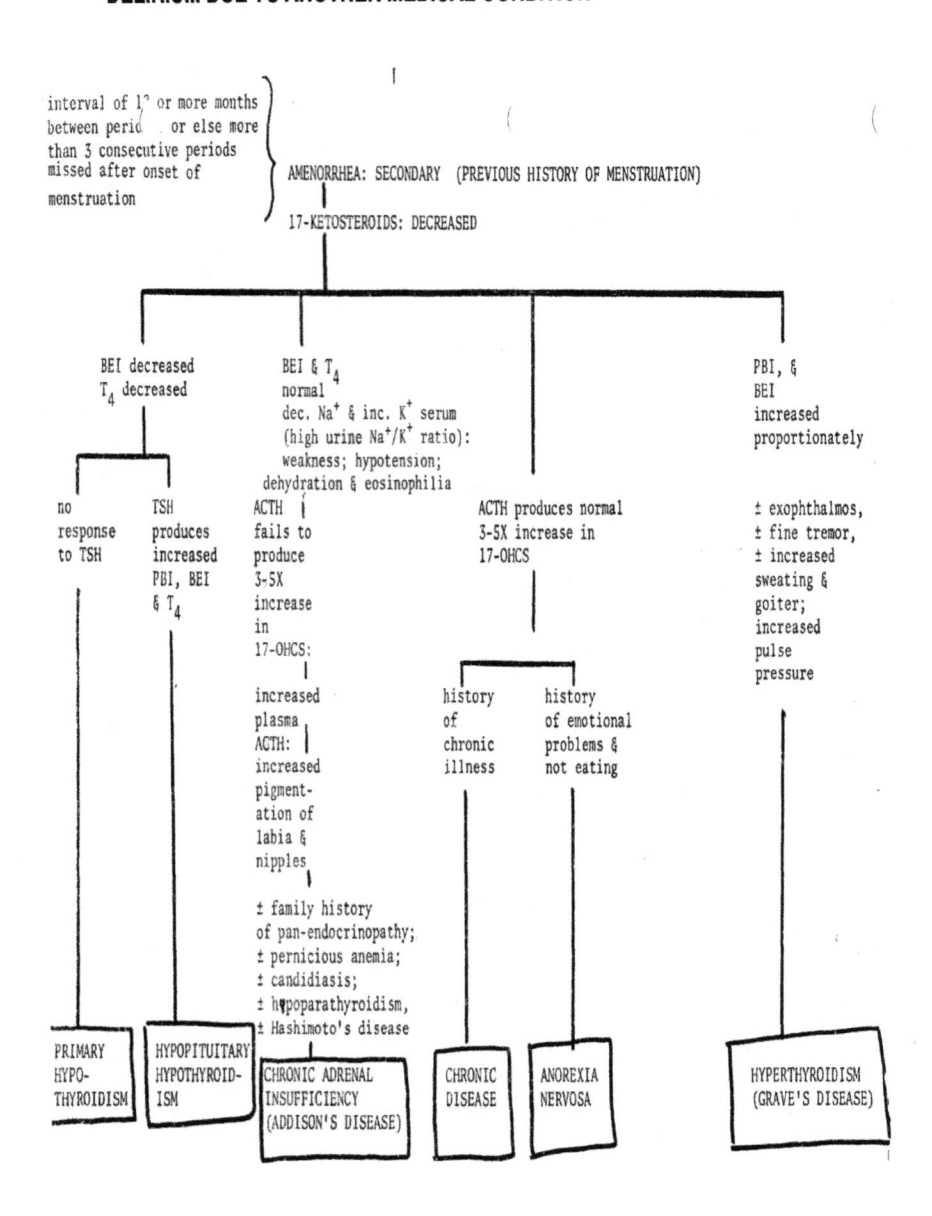

interval of 12 or more months between periods, or else more than 3 consecutive periods missed after onset of menstruation } AMENORRHEA: SECONDARY (PREVIOUS HISTORY OF MENSTRUATION)

17-KETOSTEROIDS: DECREASED

- **BEI decreased, T_4 decreased**
  - no response to TSH → **PRIMARY HYPOTHYROIDISM**
  - TSH produces increased PBI, BEI & T_4 → **HYPOPITUITARY HYPOTHYROIDISM**

- **BEI & T_4 normal; dec. Na^+ & inc. K^+ serum (high urine Na^+/K^+ ratio): weakness; hypotension; dehydration & eosinophilia**
  - ACTH fails to produce 3-5X increase in 17-OHCS:
  - increased plasma ACTH:
  - increased pigmentation of labia & nipples
  - ± family history of pan-endocrinopathy; ± pernicious anemia; ± candidiasis; ± hypoparathyroidism, ± Hashimoto's disease
  → **CHRONIC ADRENAL INSUFFICIENCY (ADDISON'S DISEASE)**

- **ACTH produces normal 3-5X increase in 17-OHCS**
  - history of chronic illness → **CHRONIC DISEASE**
  - history of emotional problems & not eating → **ANOREXIA NERVOSA**

- **PBI, & BEI increased proportionately**
  - ± exophthalmos, ± fine tremor, ± increased sweating & goiter; increased pulse pressure
  → **HYPERTHYROIDISM (GRAVE'S DISEASE)**

DELIRIUM DUE TO ANOTHER MEDICAL CONDITION

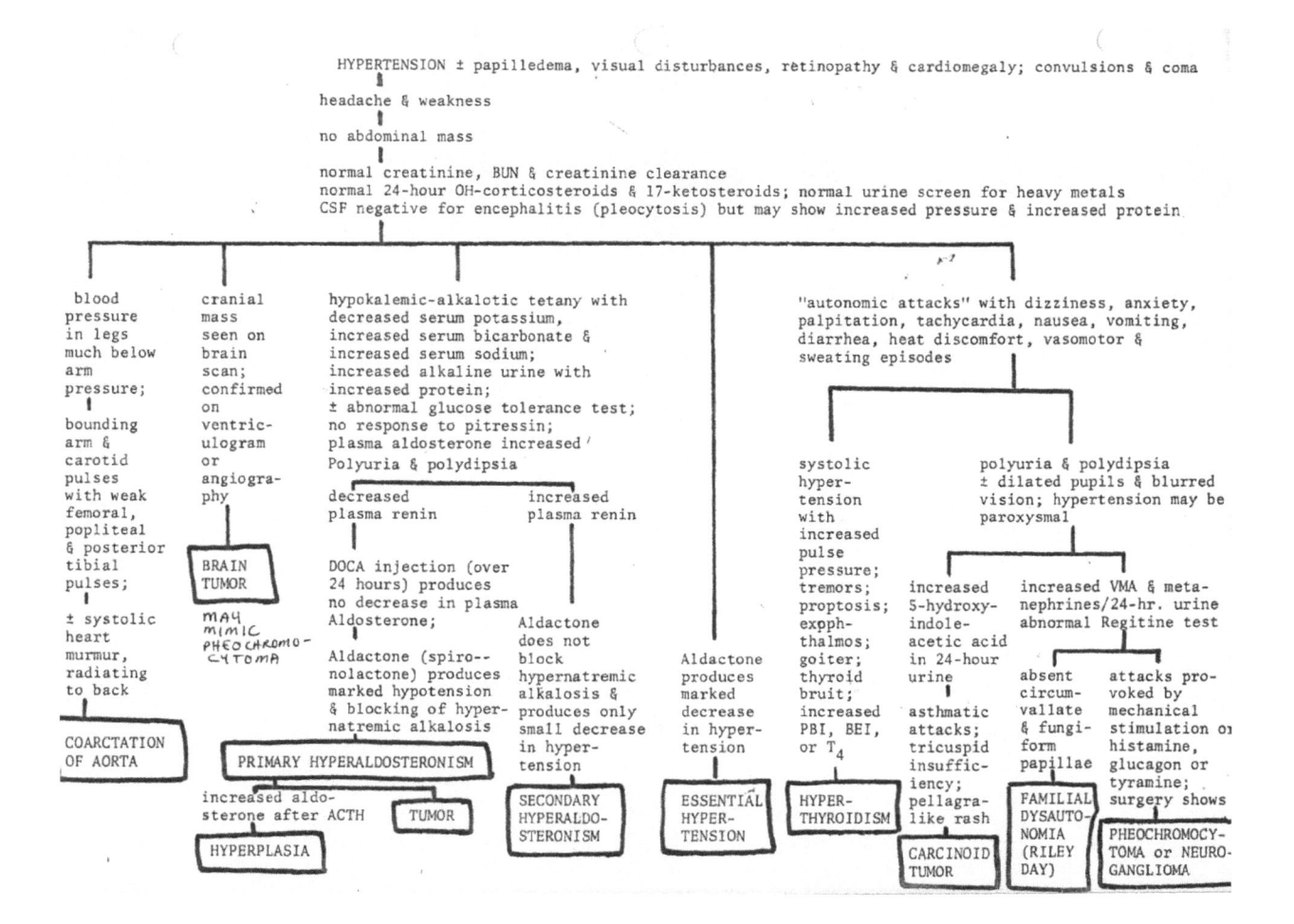

HYPERTENSION ± papilledema, visual disturbances, retinopathy & cardiomegaly; convulsions & coma
↑
headache & weakness
↑
no abdominal mass
↑
normal creatinine, BUN & creatinine clearance
normal 24-hour OH-corticosteroids & 17-ketosteroids; normal urine screen for heavy metals
CSF negative for encephalitis (pleocytosis) but may show increased pressure & increased protein

- **blood pressure in legs much below arm pressure;** bounding arm & carotid pulses with weak femoral, popliteal & posterior tibial pulses; ± systolic heart murmur, radiating to back → **COARCTATION OF AORTA**

- **cranial mass seen on brain scan; confirmed on ventriculogram or angiography** → **BRAIN TUMOR** — MAY MIMIC PHEOCHROMOCYTOMA

- **hypokalemic-alkalotic tetany with decreased serum potassium, increased serum bicarbonate & increased serum sodium; increased alkaline urine with increased protein; ± abnormal glucose tolerance test; no response to pitressin; plasma aldosterone increased / Polyuria & polydipsia**
  - decreased plasma renin → DOCA injection (over 24 hours) produces no decrease in plasma Aldosterone; Aldactone (spironolactone) produces marked hypotension & blocking of hypernatremic alkalosis → **PRIMARY HYPERALDOSTERONISM**
    - increased aldosterone after ACTH → **HYPERPLASIA**
    - TUMOR
  - increased plasma renin → Aldactone does not block hypernatremic alkalosis & produces only small decrease in hypertension → **SECONDARY HYPERALDOSTERONISM**

- Aldactone produces marked decrease in hypertension → **ESSENTIAL HYPERTENSION**

- **"autonomic attacks" with dizziness, anxiety, palpitation, tachycardia, nausea, vomiting, diarrhea, heat discomfort, vasomotor & sweating episodes**
  - systolic hypertension with increased pulse pressure; tremors; proptosis; exophthalmos; goiter; thyroid bruit; increased PBI, BEI, or T_4 → **HYPERTHYROIDISM**
  - increased 5-hydroxyindoleacetic acid in 24-hour urine; asthmatic attacks; tricuspid insufficiency; pellagra-like rash → **CARCINOID TUMOR**
  - polyuria & polydipsia ± dilated pupils & blurred vision; hypertension may be paroxysmal
    - absent circumvallate & fungiform papillae → **FAMILIAL DYSAUTONOMIA (RILEY DAY)**
    - increased VMA & metanephrines/24-hr. urine abnormal Regitine test; attacks provoked by mechanical stimulation or histamine, glucagon or tyramine; surgery shows → **PHEOCHROMOCYTOMA or NEUROGANGLIOMA**

DELIRIUM DUE TO ANOTHER MEDICAL CONDITION: Metabolic Acidosis

FAINTING,, COMA; HYPOMANIC; "MELTDOWNS"; UNEXPLAINABLE CONFUSIONAL STATES/ RAPID MOOD CYCLING

+/- SEIZURES

URINALYSIS:
 __for pH & ketones
 __test for reducing substances: if positive, __ get chromatography to distinguish which sugar is present
 __ sample for amino acids & organic acids (CAUTION: ORGANIC ACIDS MAY BE NORMAL IN MEDIUM CHAIN Acyl-CoA Dehydrogenase deficiency)
 do SEQUENCING HFI gene for hereditary fructose intolerance after urinalysis for reducing substances (not routine test for glucose)

BLOOD
 __Serum Glucose
 __ammonia
 electrolytes
 __lactate & pyruvate
 triglyceride
 __cholesterol
 __uric acid
 __transaminases
 __creatine kinase

DO urinary organic acid analysis whenever there is:
 __Unexplained metabolic acidosis,
 __hypoglycemia,
 ketonuria,
 __lactic acidosis
 __hyperammonemia,
 __clinical signs of systemic intoxication, __ encephalopathy
 __unexplained neurological disorders,
 __multisystem failure or
 __hepatic dysfunction.

DEFECTS OF CARBOHYDRATE METABOLISM; DEFECTS OF AMINO ACID METABOLISM; ORGANIC ACID DISORDERS; DEFECTS OF FATTY ACID METABOLISM;

Ch. 5: AMNESTIC DISORDERS

The **signature impairment** of Amnestic Disorders is the **difficulty with the retroactive retrieval and proactive storage** of memories - causing a seemingly rapid decay of data to which the victim has been exposed. This impairment is tested as soon as the patient arrives for the mental status examination using the Luria **"10-word" Test for Intermediate Memory"**. The patient is tested every 5 minutes for the first 15 minutes to obtain a highest score. At each 5-minute interval, the patient is taught again the words which were missed. An average person can remember **7-words (+/-2) by the 20-minute recall**. Someone with an Amnestic Disorder will usually score less than 5 words at that time. The classic example is a victim of a **M**otor **V**ehicle **A**ccident which produces a **concussion** where severity of the injury can be estimated by the amount of retrograde amnesia (the memory retained prior to the head injury). Oftentimes the victim has **no** recall of the actual accident occurrence (if unconsciousness exceeded 30 minutes). In the even more serious Traumatic Brain Injury cases, future risk is often stratified by the Glascow Coma Scale where a **medium-risk** scores 8: there is a brief loss of consciousness, a brief post-traumatic amnesia, some confusion, headache and vomiting at the emergency room examination. **High-risk** patients, however, show head or neck trauma, prolonged confusion and amnesia - giving little history of the traumatic blow & preceding events. They may show post-traumatic seizures or have a history of epilepsy.

Neuropsychologist Alexander Luria, who studied brain-injured soldiers in World War II, developed the above unique auditory **Intermediate Memory Test**. Intermediate memory is scored at 20 minutes and at 45 minutes. Thus a patient who recalled 8 words at the 20 minute point but only 4 words at the 45 minute point would be showing a good **intermediate** memory but also showing an impaired **REMOTE memory recall** of only 50% at 45 minutes. Psychologists use the Wechsler Delayed Logical Memory Test to assess intermediate memory function.

In Amnestic Disorders, besides the intact **immediate memory** recall, most of the other cognitive functions (except for the signature intermediate memory impairment) may appear to show only minor difficulties. If there is an apparent defect in emotional expressions, it does not reflect the patients own experience or perception of emotion. There is preservation of willed action as well.

When the brain's limbic system is impaired, this special memory loss occurs - which neurologist Raymond Adams, M.D. described in his textbook as "Axial Amnesia" but which DSM-IV and the DSM-5 have termed **Amnestic Disorder**. Severe Major Depressive Disorder (seen in "Pseudodementia") and sometimes very severe anxiety as well as "normal aging" in many people can impact the retrieval of stored memories and affect hippocampal function. Mimicking an incipient dementia, we often see in the elderly an **A**ge **A**ssociated **M**emory **I**mpairment (AAMI) exemplified by difficulty retrieving familiar names or information which will later "percolate" into memory when the anxiety state lessens or attention improves.

Although semantic memory is usually intact, Amnestic Disorder can impair "contextual" memories - for example:: "When did this happen?"; "How did this happen?"; "Where did this happen?". The limbic system has a large storage capacity lasting minutes to years when not damaged. But it does show slow accessibility and lability of maintenance when distractions are prominent. Patients are usually capable of deducing abstractions on the "Proverbs Test" if they previously had that capacity.

Thiamine deficiency (whether through chronic alcoholism, chemotherapy, chronic dialysis, inflammatory gastric disease, eating disorders or malnutrition) damages parts of the brain and especially impairs "the Limbic System". The most classic example is the Korsakoff's Syndrome which initially may be associated with only intermediate/recent memory losses (and which at first may be coupled with a compensatory **confabulation** - where the patient automatically details answers to questions (possibly with a free-floating-anxiety-driven response) which has little connection to the **facts**! See:

F10.26 Alcohol Major Neurocognitive Disorder with alcohol use; amnestic-confabulatory type; and

F10.97 Alcohol Major Neurocognitive Disorder without alcohol use; amnestic-confabulatory type.

Limbic damage eventually leads to **proactive memory loss** which begins from the onset of limbic illness or injury and which will be evidenced in a significant "long-term memory loss" from the time of the severe damage. This may cause a diagnostic confusion often to the clinician attempting to separate the dysfunctions. Possibly related to B vitamin/ thiamine depletion is what neurologists have termed the Remote Effects of Carcinoma (now termed **Paraneoplastic Encephalopathy**) and given the ICD-10-CM coding:

G13.1 Other systemic atrophy primarily affecting the Central Nervous System in Neoplastic Disease.

To make this diagnosis, there should be evidence of cancer occurring within 5 years of noting the neurological symptoms or one must search for paraneoplastic antibodies such as: *Amphipysin; CV2; Hu; Ma2 and Ri*. AN MRI scan of the brain might show bilateral MRI FLAIR or T2. An EEG with history of seizures may show bilateral involvement of the temporal lobes, or slow-wave activity.

Neurologists recognize a condition associated with epilepsy called Transient Epileptic Amnesia identified by recurrent episodes of a transient global amnesia which may be present when waking from sleep, may be associated with olfactory hallucinations, and with automatisms such as mouth-twitching and eye-blinking. An EEG with nasopharyngeal leads and sleep tracings (during an interictal period) may identify the focal source of partial/ focal seizures when not in status - and these episodes may respond to anticonvulsant medications. They are sometimes associated with atrophy of the hippocampus which may be seen on MRI scan. See:

G45.4 Transient Global Amnesia

In almost all stages of memory loss there may be impairments of orientation during the confusional states - with difficulties recalling the date, place, and circumstances for the evaluation. Following a stroke in the non-dominant hemisphere (I 63.9) visual processing deficits may impair recognition of oneself in the mirror and there may be **neglect** of the opposite side of one's body called *anosognosia* (unawareness of one's impairments) - but **not loss of one's identity** *per se*. However, except for cases of malingering, one rarely is disoriented "to self" - - - forgetting whom one is. Nevertheless, in **dissociative fugue states** there **may** be extensive retrograde amnesia as well as loss of one's personal identity. The ICD-10-CM codes are:

F44.0   Dissociative Amnesia; and

F44.82 Dissociative Identity Disorder

Focal seizures after status may show such problems.

Finally, no discussion of amnestic disorder is complete without the evaluation for **encephalitis** and **encephalopathies.** At the top of the list is Limbic Encephalitis - often caused by the Herpes Simplex Type I virus; but sometimes caused by Herpes Simplex Type VI. (Autoantibodies for the virus might be identified in the CSF fluid). The onset might be subacute (<4 years), or there may a more gradual onset with seizures, recent memory losses, and psychiatric symptoms. MRI / SPECT Scan or PET scan should show the limbic involvement. Any of the multiple encephalopathies must be considered in the differential diagnoses of Delirium Due to Another Medical Condition or causing an amnestic disorder at some stage of their presentation. Among these is the MELAS syndrome (E88.41) which is **M**itochondrial **E**ncephalopathy **L**actic **A**cidosis and **S**troke-like-episodes. (After normal childhood developmental milestones, there may appear a myopathy with muscle weakness or pain; anorexia/ vomiting; headaches and convulsions with transient ischemic attacks (T.I.A.) and migraine-like headaches. Because they usually show a lactic acidosis, they would usually be identified in the initial confusional state of **delirium**. Continuous episodes lead to brain damage to the point of dementia).

Sudden onset of limbic disease suggests an emboss or infarct to the anterior communicating artery of the brain - for instance as in Sickle Cell Disease. The onset may seem rapid in paraneoplastic dementia or "Remote Effect of Carcinoma".

Episodic spells of limbic impairment may suggest Vertebro-Basilar Artery migraine or T.I.A. or vertebrobasilar compression from cervical osteophytes as well as vertebrobasilar artery Fibromuscular Dysplasia.

Transient limbic impairment may follow a Traumatic Brain Injury ("Post-Traumatic Amnesia") - r unilateral infarct of the left hippocampal region as well as early onset of Korsakoff's Syndrome - or thiamine deficit. (Failure to provide intravenous thiamine then has sometimes precipitated pontine myelinolysis and death in such cases).

The gradual onset of limbic disease suggests Korsakoff's Syndrome, brain tumors or abscess with bitemporal involvement or a colloid cyst of the Third Ventricle.

CH. 6: DEMENTIA & NCDs

DSM-5 has classified neurocognitive disorders into three useful categories:

1. DELIRIUM - the acute onset of a confusional state evidenced by significant **impairment** in attention or **Immediate Memory**.

2. AMNESTIC DISORDERS - the variable onset of **Recent / Intermediate Memory Dysfunction**.

3. MAJOR / MILD NEUROCOGNITIVE DISORDERS of predominantly **Long-Term Memories**, behaviors, and skills **which had been previously acquired.**

These were previously categorized as the "**dementias**" whose probable causes are now codified as:

DSM-5 CODE	**DIAGNOSIS**
F02.8X	___ ALZHEIMER'S DISEASE
	___ LEWY BODY DISEASE
	___ TRAUMATIC BRAIN INJURY
G31.09 [F02.81]	___ FRONTOTEMPORAL LOBAR DEGENERATION with behavioral disturbance
G31.09 [F02.80]	___ FRONTOTEMPORAL LOBAR DEGENERATION without behavioral disturbance
F01.5x [F02.81]	___ NCD secondary to VASCULAR DISEASE
B20 [F02.80]	___ HIV ASSOCIATED NEUROCOGNITIVE DISORDER
A81.9 [F02.81]	___ PRION ASSOCIATED NEUROCOGNITIVE DISORDER

G20   [F02.80] ___   PARKINSON'S DISEASE DEMENTIA

G10   [F02.81] ___   HUNTINGTON'S DISEASE DEMENTIA

F10.27 [F08.81] ___   ALCOHOL NCD with use; non-amnestic-confabulatory type

F10.97 [F02.81] ___   ALCOHOL NCD without use; non-amnestic-confabulatory type

F10.26 [F02.81] ___   ALCOHOL NCD with use; amnestic-confabulatory type

F10.96 [F02.81] ___   ALCOHOL NCD without use; amnestic-confabulatory type

(The post-script above ".80" implies "without behavioral disturbance" while the postscript ".81" implies "with behavioral disturbance"). The general rule of thumb is to precede the neurocognitive code with the specific ICD-10-CM code for the specific medical illness which is likely responsible for the neurocognitive disturbance.

It should now be apparent that most illnesses associated with amnestic disorders and impairments of the hippocampus which stores and retrieves memories will be **followed** by an anterograde amnesia - which, if permanent, will block the brain's capacity to lay down new memories and therefore which will cause a loss of detailed **"long-term" memories** from the time of illness at the hippocampal-limbic level. Now, as we review the Major and Mild neurocognitive Disorders familiarized as the "dementias", we will also see what **specific damage to various cortical areas** can add to the disappearance of long-term memories, behaviors, skills and information. Such generalized and diffuse cortical damage, we are now aware, is the cause of **generalized behavioral and developmental losses** as well.

Alzheimer's Disease, the prototype dementia, is recognized by impairments of long-term memories and capacities which occur in an "onion-ring" deterioration. Retrieval of the most recent memories is unavailable, then the next strata of memories is unretrievable, so that eventually the patient believes he/she is "living in the childhood years". Possibly the best screening test for **remote memory ability** is the **recall at 1 hour** (the end of the mental status examination) of the Luria "10-word Test" - which was used for Intermediate Memory. The clinician is looking for **deterioration** in capacity to retain memory. It has been shown that if Intermediate Memory at 15 minutes is an "8" and deteriorates to a "4" by 60 minutes, there is significant damage in remote memory capacity. Additionally, one then gives "hints" (see Page 123 - Long-Term Memory Testing) to see if this memory improves. In Alzheimer's Disease, there is characteristically **no improvement** after the hints are given. Also, on the **Set Test** for **"FACTS"** ("Name 10 Flowers; 10 Animals; 10 Colors; 10 Towns or cities"), Alzheimer patients score 29 or less out of the possible 40 points. All types of data can be lost including awareness, orientation, attention/ concentration, persistence capacity/drive, verbal semantic/ contextual reasoning and problem solving; visual processing of symbols, letter, patterns and processing speed; emotional and body language assessment; theory of mind (recognition of thoughts and feelings of others who are outside oneself); and insight as well as judgment. Speech and retrieval which should be specific, syntactic, abstract, descriptive, coherent and profuse may all be impaired in this dementia process.

Incipient dementia may be recognized by a decreased capacity to postpone gratification for achieving one's goals or by a decreased tolerance of frustrations. Such patients show more difficulty recovering from "life's failures" - such as loss of occupation or funds. These patients show decreased capacity to utilize effective and modulated defense mechanisms (such as suppression, humor, anticipation, altruism and sublimation). There is often a decreased energy and enthusiasm as well as a decreased creativity and task completion.

In the later stages of dementia, we see more impairment of judgment, orientation, and calculation abilities. The MAZE escape tests and clock-drawing at specific times - becomes very impaired. The recall of the "10-Word Test" will be below 50%. Affect may appear dull or flat or there may be mood lability and reactive anxiety at earlier stages at the realization of one's lost capacities. Fatigue is common. The PET scan classically reveals biparietal hypometabolism. We now have blood tests available to detect the Amyloid Beta 40/42 ratio and APOE genotypes. Most young people prefer not to know "they will probably develop Alzheimer's."

In other patients who present with dementia symptoms but who show an **improvement** when given hints on the Luria "10-Word Test" after 45 minutes, one might look for symptoms of Lewy Body Dementia or of Parkinson's Disease with Dementia (which often shows Lewy Bodies on autopsy). In Lewy Body Dementia, if Parkinson symptoms are present, they appear **after one year** of dementia symptoms. This Lewy Body dementia shows hypoperfusion of the occipital lobes on a SPECT Scan of the brain and is characterized by "acting out one's dreams" - a Rapid Eye Movement Sleep Disorder - recognized on polysomnography during a sleep study. These patients are often experiencing visual hallucinations and might seem to be showing "schizophrenic-like" symptoms.

Parkinson's Disease with Dementia is often associated with Lewy Body inclusions and may **develop dementia after 1 year** from the onset of Parkinson's symptoms such as resting, gross postural tremor of the head/neck/distal extremities or "cogwheel rigidity of extremities" and/or bradykinesia/ mask-like facies. They may also show an active voluntary movement "kinetic" tremor at the completion of a goal-directed motor activity, i.e. an "intention tremor". There may be "pillrolling" motor activity of the fingers as well.

Neurologists often subdivide FrontoTemporal Dementia into three groups depending on which area of the central nervous system degeneration appears first:

1. "PICK'S DISEASE" - the Behavioral Variety of FTD which shows predominantly a loss of social inhibitions. (These are the patients who are caught walking naked in public, for example).

2. SEMANTIC FTD - recognized by the patient's **impaired comprehension of language** and confusion at what other people are trying to tell them; and finally

3. PROGRESSIVE NON-FLUENT APHASIA - where the patient loses one's ability to **speak fluently**.

Unlike the Alzheimer patients, these patients may retain the capacity to "Draw-A-Clock" at the appropriate time and to negotiate their ambient environment without "getting lost". Striatal and orbitofrontal atrophy may also be associated with bizarre eating habits (such as gorging or taking food off the plates of other diners). On neurological examination there is often a primitive "frontal lobe release-sign" such as the Palmomental Reflex. All Neurocognitive Disorders make completion of tasks / "persistence" impaired.

The Behavioral Form of FTD might be diagnosed in vivo by a **F**luro**D**eoxy**G**lucose **P**ositron **E**mmision **T**omography scan which might show frontal and anterior temporal and ventromedial prefrontal cortex hypometabolism.

Vascular dementia may typically lose language functions later. They may show signs of pseudo-bulbar palsy such as emotional lability (unwanted and uncontrolled laughing or weeping) with difficulty controlling facial and tongue movements and slow, slurred speech. There might be difficulty swallowing and a brisk jaw jerk. Personality changes come in the later decades as well as loss of empathy which may be significant. MRI scan reveals "scattered white spots" or islands of vascular damage.

Like a ringing bell which strikes its shell both forwards and backwards, the hippocampus is damaged in head injuries in a "contracoup" response - damaging the side opposite the blow force. What follows with each blow is a progressive impairment in storing and retrieving memories. Although this might initially be detected as an amnestic disorder in athletes or soldiers continuously exposed to blows and explosive forces, it often goes unrecognized until such patients start showing emotional lability such as rage outbursts and suicidal depressions and then long-term memory and retrieval impairments. Such is the case with Post-Concussion Syndrome:

F07.81 [F02.81] Chronic Traumatic Encephalopathy.

We thus enter the category of **Neurocognitive Disorders Due to Another Medical Condition**. This category will then include a variety of disorders ranging from:

NEUROCOGNITIVE DISORDERS DUE TO ANOTHER MEDICAL CONDITION

1. BRAIN TUMORS & CNS A-V Malformations;

2. CARDIOVASCULAR DISORDERS: such as Lacunar State/ stroke/ Carotid Stenosis; S/P Hypoxic/Anoxic events;

3. DEMYELINATING STATES such as Multiple Sclerosis;

4. ENDOCRINOPATHIES: such as Adrenal Insufficiency (Addison's Disease); parathyroid/ pituitary/ thyroid disorders (especially occult hypothyroidism);

5. HYDROCEPHALUS: occult "Normal Pressure Hydrocephalus"; and increased pressure hydrocephalus;

6. IMMUNE DISORDERS: such as Systemic Lupus Erythematosus;

7. INFECTIOUS DISORDERS: such as neurosyphilis and measles (Subacute Sclerosing Panencephalitis);

8. METABOLIC DISORDERS: such as KUF'S Adrenoleukodystrophy, Pantothenate-Kinase-Associated NCD, Wilson's Disease; Pyruvate-Dehydrogenase Deficiency ("Leigh's Disease), Globoid Cell Leukodystrophy (Krabbe's Disease), Aminoacid Disorders, etc.

9. ORGAN FAILURE: such as hepatic cirrhosis/ hyperammonemia; and renal failure/ uremia; dialysis/ azotemia

10. TRAUMA: such as Chronic Traumatic Encephalopathy;

11. VITAMIN DEFICIENCY: such as B12-deficient Subacute Combined Degeneration & Wernicke's Encephalopathy secondary to thiamine deficiency.

LONG-TERM Memory Testing

HOW TO USE: USING THE 45 MINUTE OR 1 HOUR RECALL, GIVE HINTS & SCORE AFTER THE HINTS WERE GIVEN.

10 WORDS AT 1 HOUR: GIVE HINT FOR ANY WORD WHICH WAS NOT RECALLED & SCORE "AFTER HINT" TOTAL.

AFTER HINT SCORE

Word	Hint	
DOG	MAN'S BEST FRIEND	_____
AXE	A TOOL USED TO CUT TREES.	
WEST	ONE OF THE 4 DIRECTIONS ON A MAP.	
EAR	A PART OF A PERSON'S FACE.	
FENCE	THIS ENCLOSES A YARD OR PARKING LOT.	
SONG	A MUSICAL MELODY.	
BOAT	A MEANS OF TRAVELING ON THE WATER	
NIGHT	A PART OF THE 24 HR DAY	
CLOCK	IT IS USED TO TELL TIME	
KEY	IT IS USED TO OPEN UP A LOCKED DOOR.	_____

SCORING: A SCORE BELOW 5 WITHOUT HINTS IS A FAILING SCORE.

IF HINTS ALLOW ADDITIONAL MEMORY POINTS, IF SCORE IS STILL BELOW 6, CONSIDER DEMENTIA SECONDARY TO FRONTOTEMPORAL DEMENTIA & LEWY BODY DEMENTIA.

EARLY DEMENTIA

Decreased Capacity to Postpone Gratification;
Decreased Frustration Tolerance & Ability to Recover from Failure;
Decreased Capacity to Utilize Effective, Modulated Defense Mechanisms;
Impaired Judgment, Orientation, Memory & Calculation Abilities;
Affect Dull or Flattened +/- Reactive Anxiety over Realization of Lost Functions

PARKINSON'S SYNDROME esp. Cogwheel RIGIDITY & resting tremor

- Hx sudden onset headache/ loss of consciousness in a person with long-sustained hypertension (esp. diastolic >120) +/- any ONE of these:
  (1) Pure motor hemiplegia;
  (2) Homolateral ataxia & crural knee paresis;
  (3) Dysarthria & clumsy hand syndrome;
  (4) Pure sensory stroke with recovery from stroke; +/- PSEUDOBULBAR PALSY (pathologic laughing/crying), small-stepped gait;
  +/- early age onset
  → **LACUNAR STATE (Arterio-vascular Dementia)**

- Loss of voluntary pursuit movements of the eyes; esp. limitation of voluntary upward gaze +/- preservation of full reflex movements initially (on "Doll's Head" maneuver; +/- resting, dystonic head posturing; ADULT ONSET esp. 6th decade; +/- inc. jaw jerk; abnormal snout/ grasp/root; +/- Pseudobulbar Palsy & UMN X, XI, XII; +/- PYRAMIDAL TRACT & CEREBELLAR dysfunction; +/- brain stem nuclei
  → **PROGRESSIVE SUPRANUCLEAR PALSY; Steele-Richardson Olszewski**

- Onset 5-th to 6th decade; falling episodes masklike facies; festinating gait.

- +/- incontinence; apnea; erectile dysfunction; dizziness; neck ache; orthostatic hypotension; dry skin dysphagia
  → **SHY-DRAGER SYNDROME**

  → **PARKINSON'S DISEASE**

- EEG shows absent/ decreased alpha activity; CT/ PEG shows increased width of sulcal markings & ventricular enlargement; esp anterior & temporal horns atrophy disuse; accumulation of amyloid plaques in typical locations
  → **ALZHEIMER'S DISEASE**

- Frontal atrophy; esp middle, inferior & anterior of superior Temporal Lobe; accumulation of Tau protein P.E.G. abn. Fluorodeoxy-glucose PET scan typical BITEMPORO-PARIETAL & POSTERIOR CINGULATE CORTICAL abnormalities
  → **FRONTO-TEMPORAL DEMENTIA "Pick's"**

- Onset @ any age; subacute course +/- seizures; Motor Weakness; Visual Imperceptions Neuronal degeneration of spinal cord & spongiform encephalopathy; slow virus
  → **CREUTZFELDT-JAKOB SYNDROME**

142

NEUROCOGNITIVE DISORDERS DIFFERENTIAL FOR "DEMENTIA"

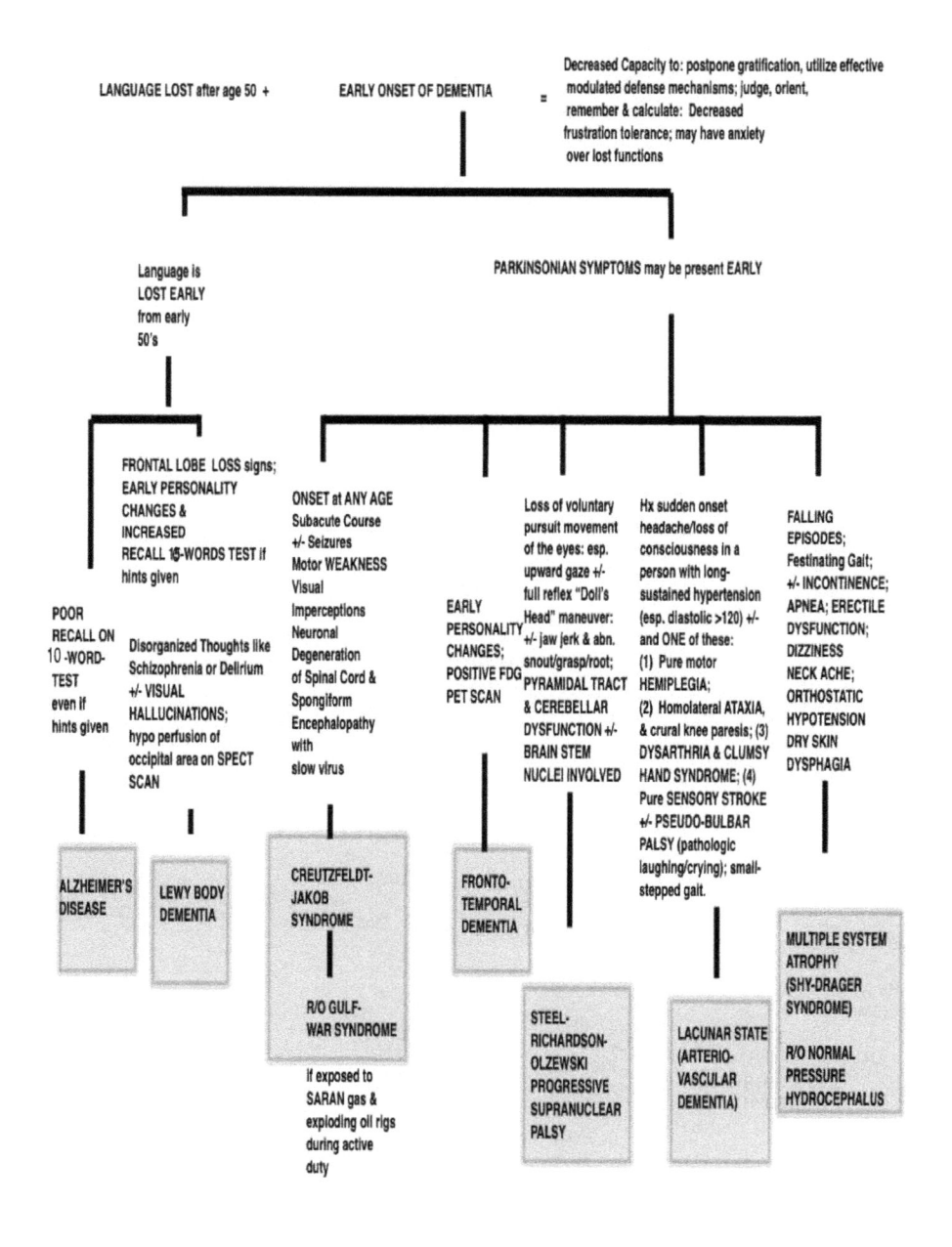

LANGUAGE LOST after age 50 + EARLY ONSET OF DEMENTIA = Decreased Capacity to: postpone gratification, utilize effective modulated defense mechanisms; judge, orient, remember & calculate; Decreased frustration tolerance; may have anxiety over lost functions

Language is LOST EARLY from early 50's

PARKINSONIAN SYMPTOMS may be present EARLY

FRONTAL LOBE LOSS signs; EARLY PERSONALITY CHANGES & INCREASED RECALL 15-WORDS TEST if hints given

- **POOR RECALL ON 10-WORD-TEST even if hints given** → **ALZHEIMER'S DISEASE**

- **Disorganized Thoughts like Schizophrenia or Delirium +/- VISUAL HALLUCINATIONS; hypo perfusion of occipital area on SPECT SCAN** → **LEWY BODY DEMENTIA**

- **ONSET at ANY AGE Subacute Course +/- Seizures Motor WEAKNESS Visual Imperceptions Neuronal Degeneration of Spinal Cord & Spongiform Encephalopathy with slow virus** → **CREUTZFELDT-JAKOB SYNDROME** → **R/O GULF-WAR SYNDROME** if exposed to SARAN gas & exploding oil rigs during active duty

- **EARLY PERSONALITY CHANGES; POSITIVE FDG PET SCAN** → **FRONTO-TEMPORAL DEMENTIA**

- **Loss of voluntary pursuit movement of the eyes: esp. upward gaze +/- full reflex "Doll's Head" maneuver; +/- jaw jerk & abn. snout/grasp/root; PYRAMIDAL TRACT & CEREBELLAR DYSFUNCTION +/- BRAIN STEM NUCLEI INVOLVED** → **STEEL-RICHARDSON-OLZEWSKI PROGRESSIVE SUPRANUCLEAR PALSY**

- **Hx sudden onset headache/loss of consciousness in a person with long-sustained hypertension (esp. diastolic >120) +/- and ONE of these: (1) Pure motor HEMIPLEGIA; (2) Homolateral ATAXIA, & crural knee paresis; (3) DYSARTHRIA & CLUMSY HAND SYNDROME; (4) Pure SENSORY STROKE +/- PSEUDO-BULBAR PALSY (pathologic laughing/crying); small-stepped gait.** → **LACUNAR STATE (ARTERIO-VASCULAR DEMENTIA)**

- **FALLING EPISODES; Festinating Gait; +/- INCONTINENCE; APNEA; ERECTILE DYSFUNCTION; DIZZINESS NECK ACHE; ORTHOSTATIC HYPOTENSION DRY SKIN DYSPHAGIA** → **MULTIPLE SYSTEM ATROPHY (SHY-DRAGER SYNDROME)** → **R/O NORMAL PRESSURE HYDROCEPHALUS**

NEUROCOGNITIVE DISORDER DUE TO LACUNAR STATE

PAST HISTORY OF T.I.A. / STROKE

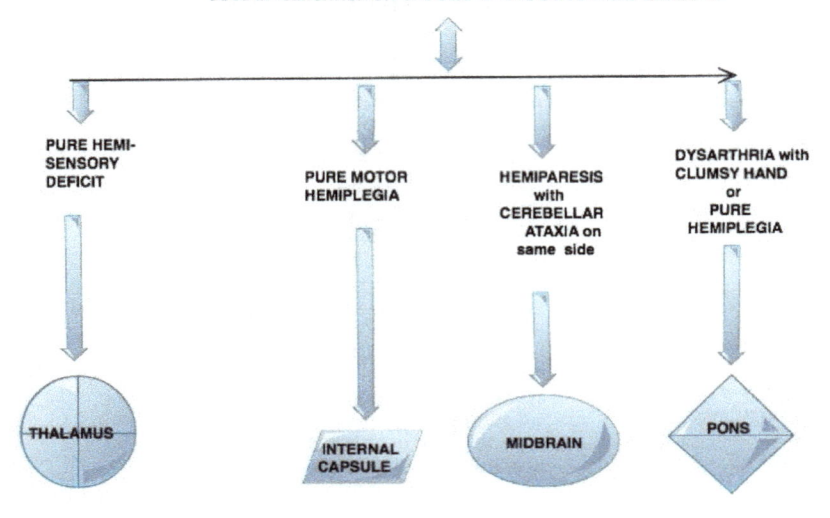

SUDDEN ONSET OF HEADACHE/ CONFUSION/ DIFFICULTY SPEAKING/ DIFFICULTY MOVING ONE'S HAND PROPERLY OR ONE SIDE OF ONE'S BODY; OR DIFFICULTY FEELING ON ONE SIDE OF ONE'S BODY/ OR "WALKING LIKE A DRUNK" (ATAXIA with Negative Romberg Test) OR LOSS OF SENSATION ON ONE SIDE OF ONE'S BODY: later DEMENTIA

- PURE HEMI-SENSORY DEFICIT → THALAMUS
- PURE MOTOR HEMIPLEGIA → INTERNAL CAPSULE
- HEMIPARESIS with CEREBELLAR ATAXIA on same side → MIDBRAIN
- DYSARTHRIA with CLUMSY HAND or PURE HEMIPLEGIA → PONS

NEUROCOGNITIVE DISORDERS DUE TO ANOTHER MEDICAL CONDITION

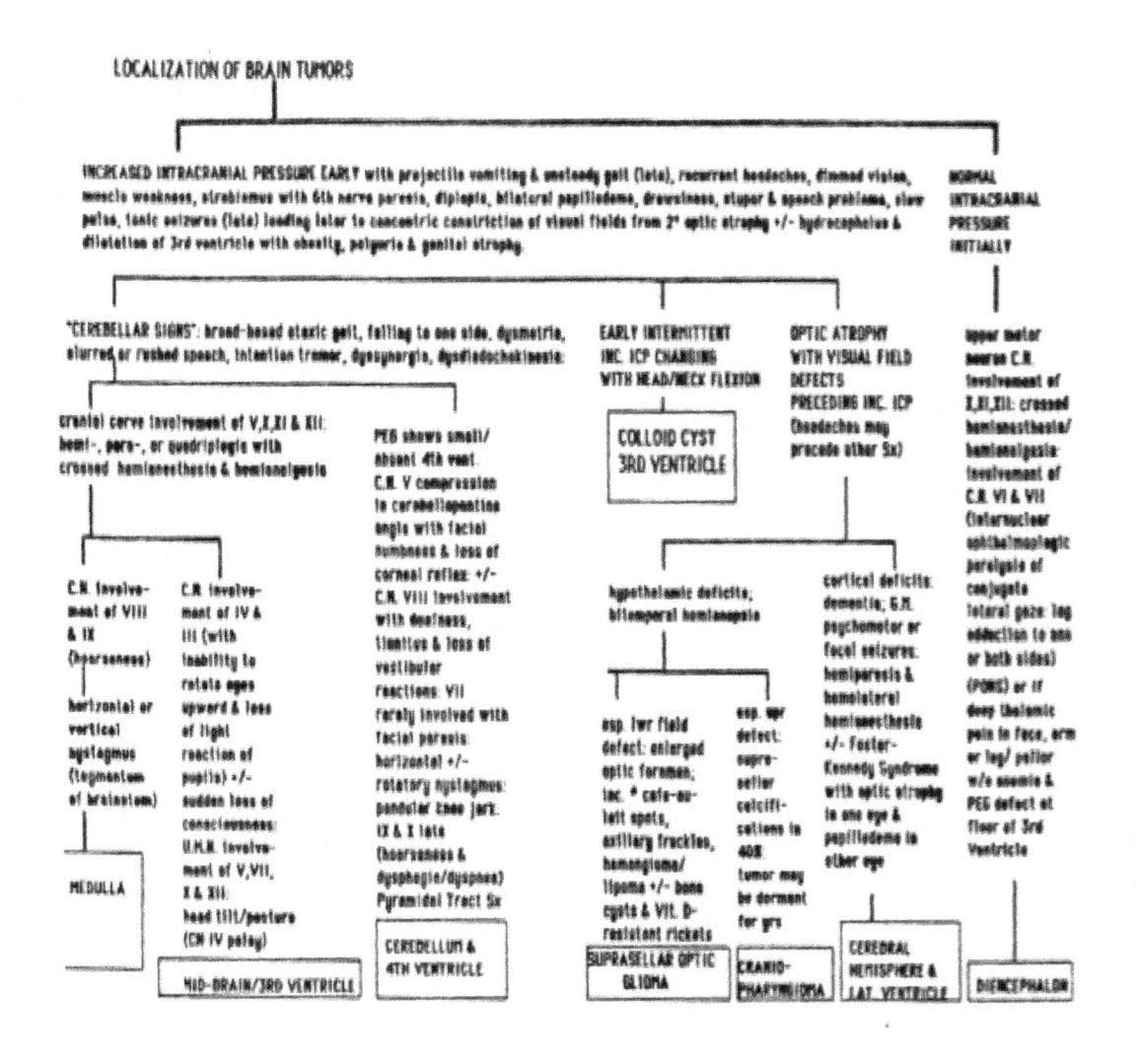

LOCALIZATION OF BRAIN TUMORS

INCREASED INTRACRANIAL PRESSURE EARLY with projectile vomiting & unsteady gait (late), recurrent headaches, dimmed vision, muscle weakness, strabismus with 6th nerve paresis, diplopia, bilateral papilledema, drowsiness, stupor & speech problems, slow pulse, tonic seizures (late) leading later to concentric constriction of visual fields from 2° optic atrophy +/- hydrocephalus & dilatation of 3rd ventricle with obesity, polyuria & genital atrophy.

NORMAL INTRACRANIAL PRESSURE INITIALLY

"CEREBELLAR SIGNS": broad-based ataxic gait, falling to one side, dysmetria, slurred or rushed speech, intention tremor, dyssynergia, dysdiadochokinesia:

EARLY INTERMITTENT INC. ICP CHANGING WITH HEAD/NECK FLEXION

OPTIC ATROPHY WITH VISUAL FIELD DEFECTS PRECEDING INC. ICP (headaches may precede other Sx)

upper motor neuron C.N. involvement of X,XI,XII: crossed hemianesthesia/hemianalgesia; involvement of C.N. VI & VII (internuclear ophthalmoplegic paralysis of conjugate lateral gaze: leg adduction to one or both sides) (PONS) or if deep thalamic pain to face, arm or leg/ pallor w/o anemia & PEG defect at floor of 3rd Ventricle

---

cranial nerve involvement of V,X,XI & XII: hemi-, para-, or quadriplegia with crossed hemianesthesia & hemianalgesia

PEG shows small/absent 4th vent. C.N. V compression in cerebellopontine angle with facial numbness & loss of corneal reflex +/- C.N. VIII involvement with deafness, tinnitus & loss of vestibular reactions: VII rarely involved with facial paresis: horizontal +/- rotatory nystagmus: pendular knee jerk: IX & X late (hoarseness & dysphagia/dyspnea) Pyramidal Tract Sx

COLLOID CYST 3RD VENTRICLE

hypothalamic deficits; bitemporal hemianopsia

cortical deficits: dementia; G.M. psychomotor or focal seizures; hemiparesis & homolateral hemianesthesia +/- Foster-Kennedy Syndrome with optic atrophy in one eye & papilledema in other eye

---

C.N. involvement of VIII & IX (hoarseness)

horizontal or vertical nystagmus (tegmentum of brainstem)

C.N. involvement of IV & III (with inability to rotate eyes upward & loss of light reaction of pupils) +/- sudden loss of consciousness; U.M.N. involvement of V,VII, X & XII: head tilt/posture (CN IV palsy)

esp. lwr field defect: enlarged optic foramen; inc. # cafe-au-lait spots, axillary freckles, hemangioma/ lipoma +/- bone cysts & Vit. D-resistant rickets

esp. upr defect: suprasellar calcifications in 40%; tumor may be dormant for yrs

MEDULLA

CEREBELLUM & 4TH VENTRICLE

MID-BRAIN/3RD VENTRICLE

SUPRASELLAR OPTIC GLIOMA

CRANIO-PHARYNGIOMA

CEREBRAL HEMISPHERE & LAT. VENTRICLE

DIENCEPHALON

DEMENTIA with PSYCHOSIS

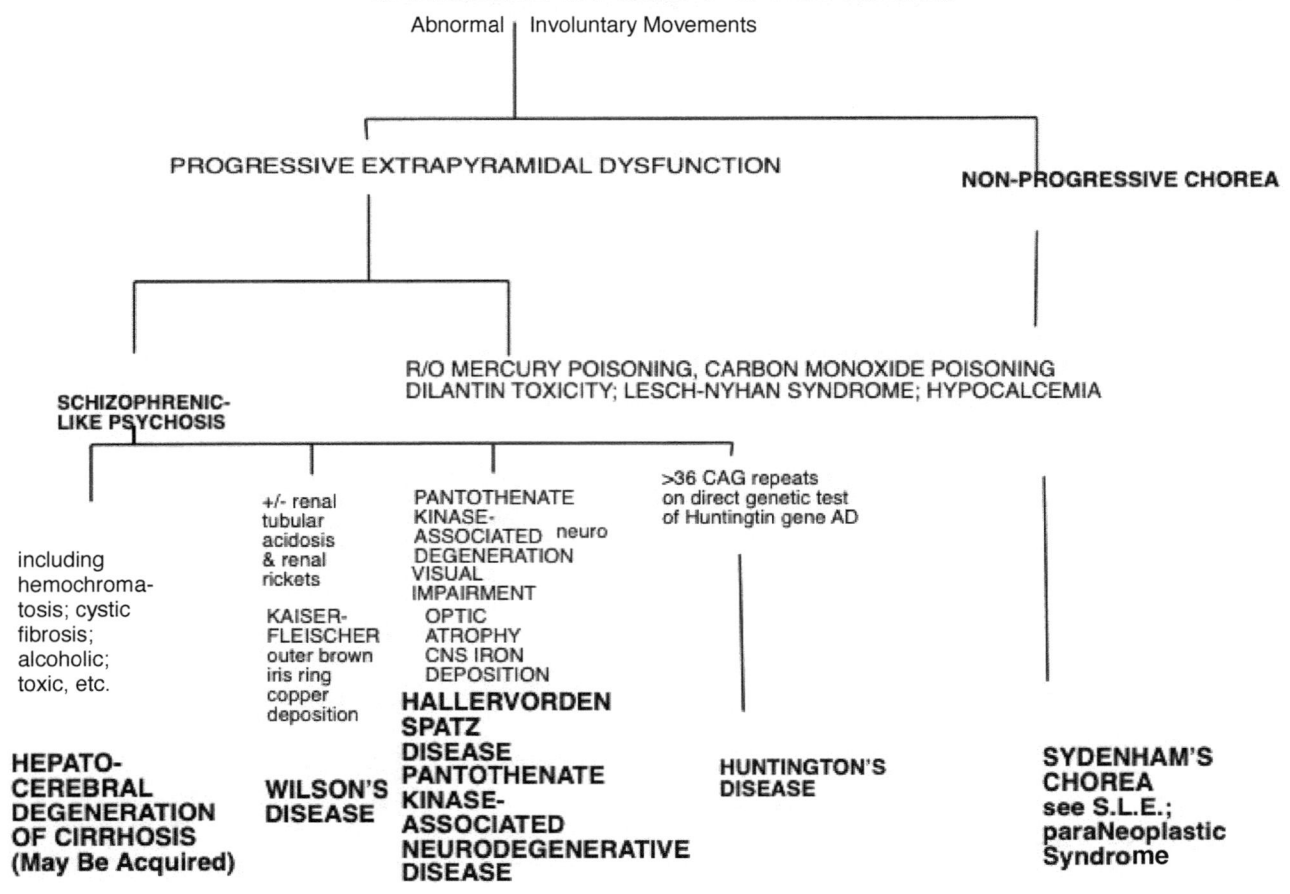

Abnormal Involuntary Movements

PROGRESSIVE EXTRAPYRAMIDAL DYSFUNCTION — NON-PROGRESSIVE CHOREA

R/O MERCURY POISONING, CARBON MONOXIDE POISONING
DILANTIN TOXICITY; LESCH-NYHAN SYNDROME; HYPOCALCEMIA

SCHIZOPHRENIC-LIKE PSYCHOSIS

including hemochromatosis; cystic fibrosis; alcoholic; toxic, etc.

HEPATO-CEREBRAL DEGENERATION OF CIRRHOSIS (May Be Acquired)

+/- renal tubular acidosis & renal rickets

KAISER-FLEISCHER outer brown iris ring copper deposition

WILSON'S DISEASE

PANTOTHENATE KINASE-ASSOCIATED neuro DEGENERATION
VISUAL IMPAIRMENT
OPTIC ATROPHY
CNS IRON DEPOSITION

**HALLERVORDEN SPATZ DISEASE
PANTOTHENATE KINASE-ASSOCIATED NEURODEGENERATIVE DISEASE**

\>36 CAG repeats on direct genetic test of Huntingtin gene AD

HUNTINGTON'S DISEASE

SYDENHAM'S CHOREA
see S.L.E.; paraNeoplastic Syndrome

DEMENTIA in Childhood with CEREBELLAR ATAXIA

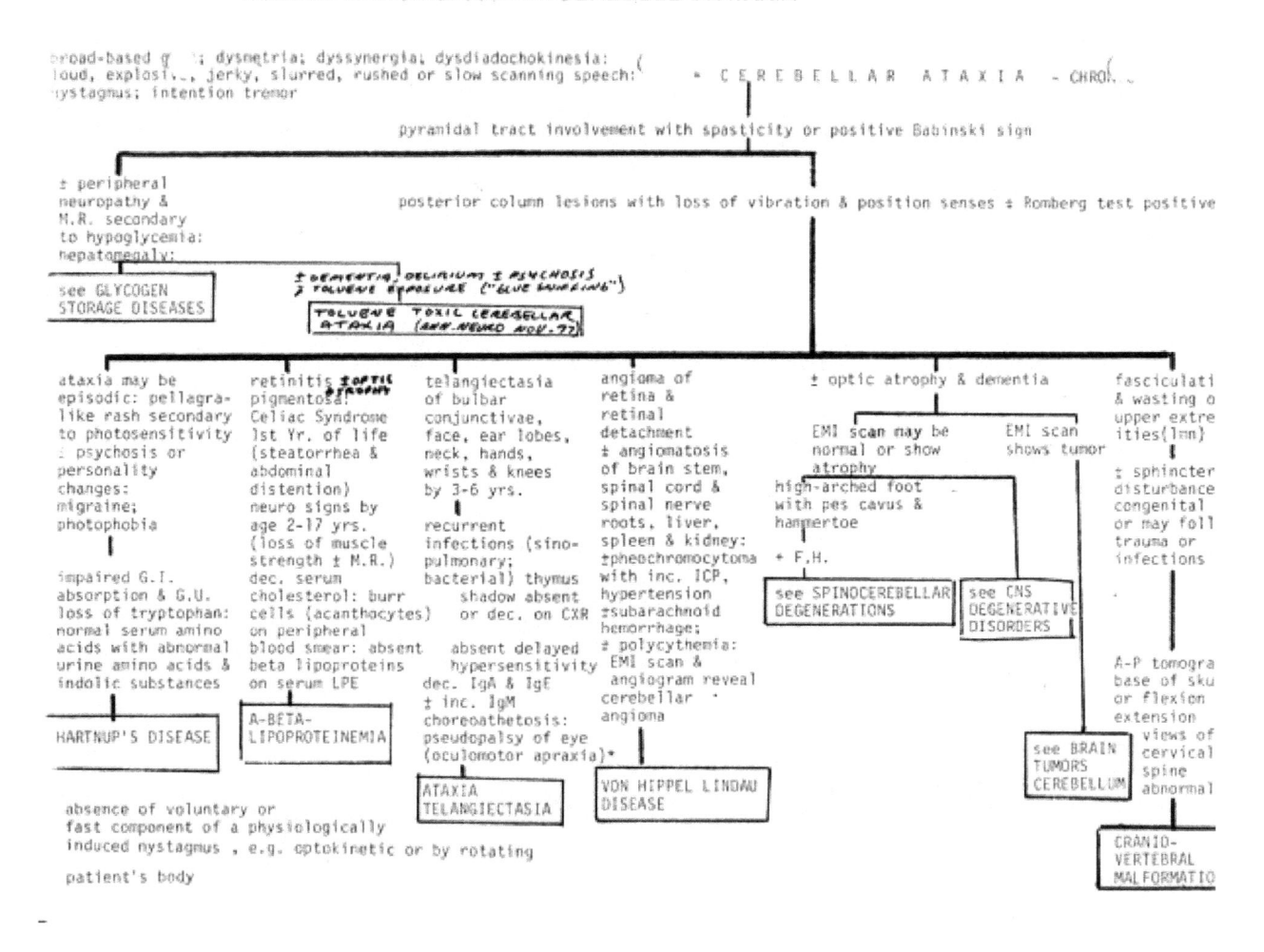

broad-based g ; dysmetria; dyssynergia; dysdiadochokinesia:
loud, explosive, jerky, slurred, rushed or slow scanning speech: = CEREBELLAR ATAXIA - CHRONIC
nystagmus; intention tremor

pyramidal tract involvement with spasticity or positive Babinski sign

± peripheral neuropathy & M.R. secondary to hypoglycemia; hepatomegaly:

posterior column lesions with loss of vibration & position senses ± Romberg test positive

see GLYCOGEN STORAGE DISEASES

± DEMENTIA, DELIRIUM ± PSYCHOSIS
± TOLUENE EXPOSURE ("GLUE SNIFFING")

TOLUENE TOXIC CEREBELLAR ATAXIA (ANN. NEURO NOV. 77)

---

ataxia may be episodic: pellagra-like rash secondary to photosensitivity: psychosis or personality changes; migraine; photophobia

impaired G.I. absorption & G.U. loss of tryptophan: normal serum amino acids with abnormal urine amino acids & indolic substances

HARTNUP'S DISEASE

---

retinitis ± OPTIC ATROPHY pigmentosa; Celiac Syndrome 1st Yr. of life (steatorrhea & abdominal distention) neuro signs by age 2-17 yrs. (loss of muscle strength ± M.R.) dec. serum cholesterol: burr cells (acanthocytes) on peripheral blood smear: absent beta lipoproteins on serum LPE

A-BETA-LIPOPROTEINEMIA

---

telangiectasia of bulbar conjunctivae, face, ear lobes, neck, hands, wrists & knees by 3-6 yrs.

recurrent infections (sino-pulmonary; bacterial) thymus shadow absent or dec. on CXR absent delayed hypersensitivity dec. IgA & IgE ± inc. IgM choreoathetosis: pseudopalsy of eye (oculomotor apraxia)*

ATAXIA TELANGIECTASIA

absence of voluntary or fast component of a physiologically induced nystagmus, e.g. optokinetic or by rotating patient's body

---

angioma of retina & retinal detachment ± angiomatosis of brain stem, spinal cord & spinal nerve roots, liver, spleen & kidney: ±pheochromocytoma with inc. ICP, hypertension ±subarachnoid hemorrhage; ± polycythemia: EMI scan & angiogram reveal cerebellar angioma

VON HIPPEL LINDAU DISEASE

± optic atrophy & dementia

EMI scan may be normal or show atrophy
high-arched foot with pes cavus & hammertoe
+ F.H.

see SPINOCEREBELLAR DEGENERATIONS

EMI scan shows tumor

see CNS DEGENERATIVE DISORDERS

see BRAIN TUMORS CEREBELLUM

---

fasciculation & wasting of upper extremities (lmn)

± sphincter disturbance congenital or may follow trauma or infections

A-P tomogram base of skull or flexion extension views of cervical spine abnormal

CRANIO-VERTEBRAL MALFORMATION

DEMENTIA in Childhood with visual field deficits +/- OPTIC ATROPHY

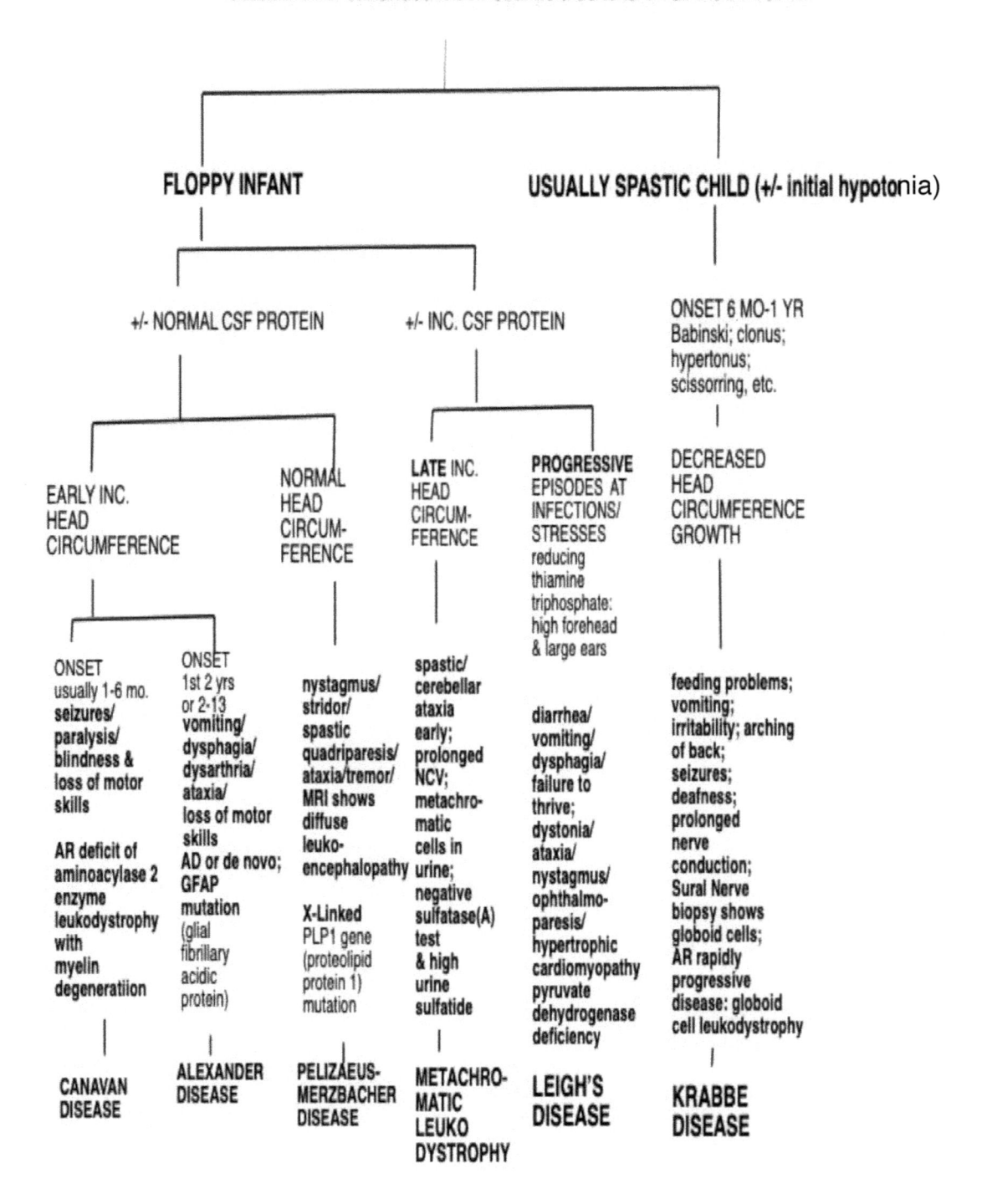

FLOPPY INFANT

+/- NORMAL CSF PROTEIN

EARLY INC. HEAD CIRCUMFERENCE

- **ONSET** usually 1-6 mo. seizures/ paralysis/ blindness & loss of motor skills

  AR deficit of aminoacylase 2 enzyme leukodystrophy with myelin degeneratiion

  → **CANAVAN DISEASE**

- **ONSET** 1st 2 yrs or 2-13 vomiting/ dysphagia/ dysarthria/ ataxia/ loss of motor skills

  AD or de novo; GFAP mutation (glial fibrillary acidic protein)

  → **ALEXANDER DISEASE**

NORMAL HEAD CIRCUMFERENCE

- nystagmus/ stridor/ spastic quadriparesis/ ataxia/tremor/ MRI shows diffuse leuko-encephalopathy

  X-Linked PLP1 gene (proteolipid protein 1) mutation

  → **PELIZAEUS-MERZBACHER DISEASE**

+/- INC. CSF PROTEIN

LATE INC. HEAD CIRCUMFERENCE

- spastic/ cerebellar ataxia early; prolonged NCV; metachromatic cells in urine; negative sulfatase(A) test & high urine sulfatide

  → **METACHROMATIC LEUKODYSTROPHY**

PROGRESSIVE EPISODES AT INFECTIONS/ STRESSES reducing thiamine triphosphate: high forehead & large ears

- diarrhea, vomiting/ dysphagia/ failure to thrive; dystonia/ ataxia/ nystagmus/ ophthalmo-paresis/ hypertrophic cardiomyopathy pyruvate dehydrogenase deficiency

  → **LEIGH'S DISEASE**

USUALLY SPASTIC CHILD (+/- initial hypotonia)

ONSET 6 MO-1 YR Babinski; clonus; hypertonus; scissorring, etc.

DECREASED HEAD CIRCUMFERENCE GROWTH

feeding problems; vomiting; irritability; arching of back; seizures; deafness; prolonged nerve conduction; Sural Nerve biopsy shows globoid cells; AR rapidly progressive disease: globoid cell leukodystrophy

→ **KRABBE DISEASE**

METABOLIC ACIDOSIS PROGRESSING TO DEMENTIA

URINALYSIS:
- for pH & ketones
- test for reducing substances: if positive, get chromatography to distinguish which sugar is present
- sample for amino acids & organic acids (CAUTION: ORGANIC ACIDS MAY BE NORMAL IN MEDIUM CHAIN Acyl-CoA Dehydrogenase deficiency)
- do SEQUENCING HFI gene for hereditary fructose intolerance after urinalysis for reducing substances (not routine test for glucose)

BLOOD
- Serum Glucose
- ammonia
- electrolytes
- lactate & pyruvate
- triglyceride
- cholesterol
- uric acid
- transaminases
- creatine kinase

DO urinary organic acid analysis whenever there is:
- Unexplained metabolic acidosis,
- hypoglycemia,
- ketonuria,
- lactic acidosis
- hyperammonemia,
- clinical signs of systemic intoxication, encephalopathy
- unexplained neurological disorders,
- multisystem failure or
- hepatic dysfunction.

Although most of these metabolic disorders such as Medium chain Acyl-CoA Dehydrogenase Deficiency and Hereditary Fructose intolerance will be recognized after the confusional states of hypoglycemia or lactic acidosis, the failure to diagnosis them earlier is another cause for metabolic dementias.

NEUROCOGNITIVE DISORDERS DUE TO ANOTHER MEDICAL CONDITION

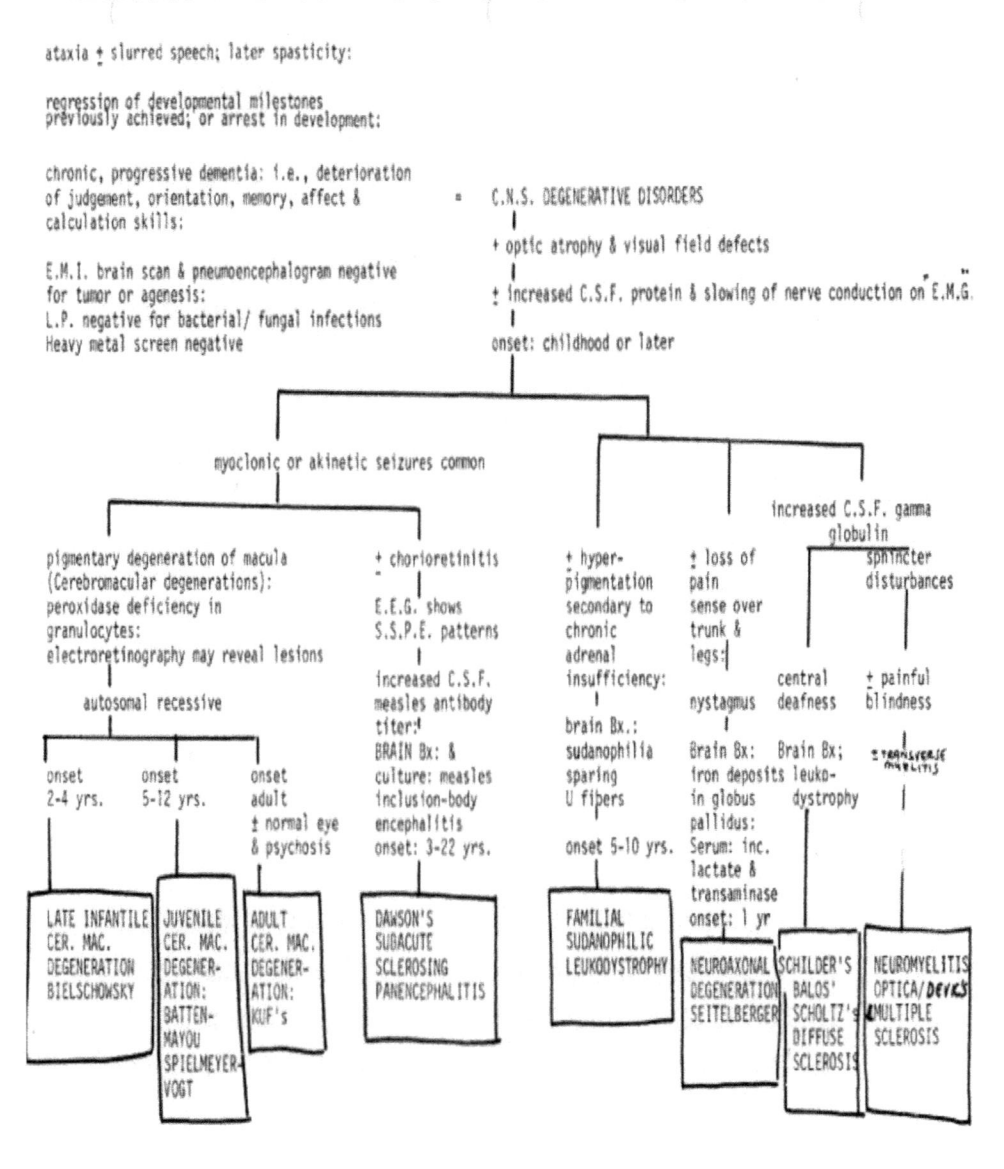

ataxia ± slurred speech; later spasticity:

regression of developmental milestones
previously achieved; or arrest in development:

chronic, progressive dementia: i.e., deterioration
of judgement, orientation, memory, affect &
calculation skills: = C.N.S. DEGENERATIVE DISORDERS

± optic atrophy & visual field defects

E.M.I. brain scan & pneumoencephalogram negative
for tumor or agenesis: ± increased C.S.F. protein & slowing of nerve conduction on E.M.G.
L.P. negative for bacterial/ fungal infections
Heavy metal screen negative   onset: childhood or later

---

myoclonic or akinetic seizures common

- pigmentary degeneration of macula (Cerebromacular degenerations): peroxidase deficiency in granulocytes: electroretinography may reveal lesions
  - autosomal recessive
    - onset 2-4 yrs. → **LATE INFANTILE CER. MAC. DEGENERATION BIELSCHOWSKY**
    - onset 5-12 yrs. → **JUVENILE CER. MAC. DEGENERATION: BATTEN-MAYOU SPIELMEYER-VOGT**
    - onset adult ± normal eye & psychosis → **ADULT CER. MAC. DEGENERATION: KUF's**

- ± chorioretinitis
  - E.E.G. shows S.S.P.E. patterns
  - increased C.S.F. measles antibody titer:
  - BRAIN Bx: & culture: measles inclusion-body encephalitis
  - onset: 3-22 yrs.
  - → **DAWSON'S SUBACUTE SCLEROSING PANENCEPHALITIS**

- ± hyper-pigmentation secondary to chronic adrenal insufficiency:
  - brain Bx.: sudanophilia sparing U fibers
  - onset 5-10 yrs.
  - → **FAMILIAL SUDANOPHILIC LEUKODYSTROPHY**

- ± loss of pain sense over trunk & legs:
  - nystagmus
  - Brain Bx: iron deposits in globus pallidus: Serum: inc. lactate & transaminase
  - onset: 1 yr
  - → **NEUROAXONAL DEGENERATION SEITELBERGER**

- increased C.S.F. gamma globulin
  - sphincter disturbances
  - central deafness
  - ± painful blindness
  - Brain Bx; leuko-dystrophy → **SCHILDER'S BALOS' SCHOLTZ'S DIFFUSE SCLEROSIS**
  - ± TRANSVERSE MYELITIS → **NEUROMYELITIS OPTICA/DEVIC'S MULTIPLE SCLEROSIS**

NEUROCOGNITIVE DISORDER DUE TO LACUNAR STATE

PAST HISTORY OF T.I.A. / STROKE

SUDDEN ONSET OF HEADACHE/ CONFUSION/ DIFFICULTY SPEAKING/ DIFFICULTY MOVING ONE'S HAND PROPERLY OR ONE SIDE OF ONE'S BODY; OR DIFFICULTY FEELING ON ONE SIDE OF ONE'S BODY/ OR "WALKING LIKE A DRUNK" (ATAXIA with Negative Romberg Test) OR LOSS OF SENSATION ON ONE SIDE OF ONE'S BODY: later DEMENTIA

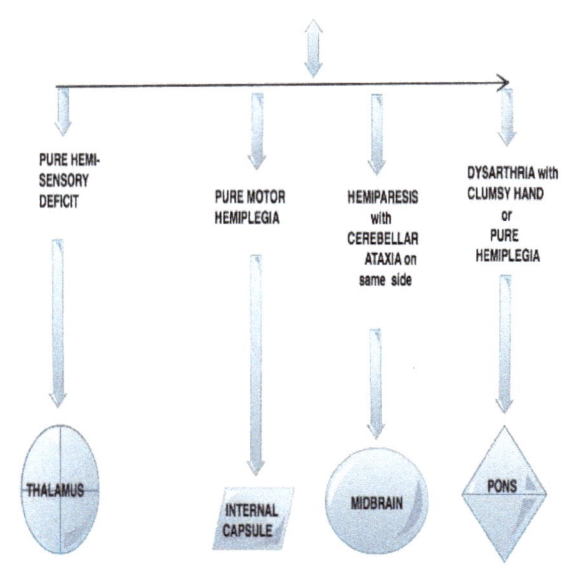

- PURE HEMI-SENSORY DEFICIT → THALAMUS
- PURE MOTOR HEMIPLEGIA → INTERNAL CAPSULE
- HEMIPARESIS with CEREBELLAR ATAXIA on same side → MIDBRAIN
- DYSARTHRIA with CLUMSY HAND or PURE HEMIPLEGIA → PONS

INDEX

INDEX TO THE NEUROCOGNITIVE DISORDERS

INDEX	PAGES
10-Word Test for Long-Term Memory	6, 32-36, 76, 78, 91, **141**
10-Word Test for Intermediate Memory - impaired	6, 78, **81**, 91, 95, 128, 129,135, 137, 149
10-Word Test improves with hints at 45-60 minutes	91, 95, 137, **141**
17-alpha-hydroxylase Deficiency adrenal hyperplasia	123
3-Step Command	**78**, 90
5-Years after neoplastic disease; neurocognitive deterioration	130, 132, **146**
A-beta-lipoproteinemia	147
Ability to count one to twenty	94
Ability to name, remember alphabet, days of week/month/yr	94
Ability to repeat 20 syllable sentence	94
Abnormal Holter Monitor with transient 3rd degree block	112, **118**
Abnorma Polysomnography	70,71,**138**
Absent pupillary/ vestibular responses Neurogenic hyperventilation	106, **111**
Abstract thinking	6,75, **77,** 78, 92, 129, 137
Acidosis - Metabolic/Respiratory Delirium	101,111, 117, 122, 126, 131, 144,148
Acidosis - Respiratory	101, 117,
acting "strange"	6
Acting out one's dreams	138
Acute Intermittent Porphyria	111, 113, 117, 123
Acyl-CoA Dehydrogenase Deficiency	117, 126, 144, 147
ADAPTABILITY/FLEXIBILITY	93
ADDISON'S DISEASE Delirium	124
Adrenal Hyperplasia/tumor; hypertensive encephalopathy	123
Adrenal insufficiency; skin pigment increased; axillary, etc.	117, 122, 124, **140,**
ADH,(INAPPROPRIATE)SYNDROME	118, 123
AFFECT/ mood	6,31, 74, 78, 89,93,107,113, 126,130,137, 150
Age-Associated-Memory-Impairment / Mild Cognitive Impairment	95, 129
ALKALOSIS METABOLIC	117
Amyloid Beta 40/42 ratio PLAQUES & APOE genotype) TESTS	137
Akinetic Seizure	44,,146
ALCOHOL NCD	136
ALEXANDER DISEASE	148
Alogia - poverty of speech/thought	8, 81
alternative reality in thought content	8, 81
Alusive thinking ("derailment")	81
Alzheimer EEG absent/dec. alpha activity; PEG inc. sulcal width	65, 85, 135, 136, 137, 141
Alzheimer's Disease: poor long-term memory even with hints	91,95, , 135, 137, 138, 142, 143
Alzheimer's Disease: Blood Tests	137,141
ambition, energy, "drive"	6, 50, 137
Amenorrhea; 17-ketosteroids decreased; Addison's	124, 125
Amenorrhea; 17-ketosteroids decreased; anorexia	124, 125
Amenorrhea; 17-ketosteroids decreased; T4/T3 GRAVE'S DISEASE	124, 125
Amenorrhea; 17-ketosteroids decreased; HYPOPITUITARY	124, 125

Amenorrhea; 17-ketosteroids decreased; HYPOTHYROIDISM	124, 125
Amenorrhea; 17-ketosteroids decreased; Addison's	124, 125
Amnestic Disorders	111, **127-134**, 135, 136, 139
Anorexia nervosa - delirium	124
Anxiety - ZUNG	29
ANXIETY DISORDERS	29, 33, 79
ARSENIC POISONING	110
Asperger Assessment in AUTISM SPECTRUM DISORDER	28-31
ATAXIA-TELANGIECTASIA SYNDROME	147
ATTENTION	9, 19, 37, 42,46, 51,71,78, 80,90,95,100,104,
ATTTUDE	74, 78, 89
Atypical Answers Roberts-2	30
AUDITORY VERBAL COMPREHENSION	94
aura (auditory sensation of buzzing)	63
aura (olfactory sensation of abhorrent smells)	36, 66
aura (tactile sensation of tingling / paresthesia)	11,29,42,52,92
aura (visual sensation) flashing lights	43, 63
AUTISM SPECTRUM DISORDERS	8, **28**-29, 89, 90, 119
Autoimmune POLYARTERITIS SJOGREN	101, 111, 117
BEHAVIOR	6,28,63,71,78,89,92,100,135,136,138,139
behavior toward others revealing mood	89
BIPOLAR DISORDER - DEPRESSED/ MIXED	63, 65, 66, 67
BIPOLAR DISORDER - MANIC	7, 20, **31**, 89, 91-94
Bipolar Mood Disorder Questionnaire - MDQ	19,20,**31**, 89, 91-94
blindness	43,84, 148, 150,
blink reflex lost	84, 85
boastfulness	89
BOTULISM	117
BRAIN/ CEREBRAL TUMORS causing DEMENTIA	101, 118,125,140, 147
BRADYCARDIA	118
caloric vestibular test abnormal	82, 102, 106
Canavan Disease	148
capacity for maintaining relationships with others	6, 51, 138-143
capacity for performing Activities of Daily Living - ADL	6, 51, 138-152
CARBON MONOXIDE POISONING/ SMOKE INHALATION	108
CARDIOVASCULAR DISORDERS causing DEMENTIA	140
carotid sinus pressure in elderly slowing heart rate	112
carotid sinus pressure in young drops B.P.	112
Carotid Artery Stenosis causing dementia	118, 119, 140
Carotid Artery FIBROMUSCULAR DYSPLASIA	119
Carotid Artery THROMBUS - with Atrial Fibrillation	119
catastrophic reaction to loss of a game or event	28-30
categorization/ conceptualization/ creativity/ interpreting	6,7,8, 94, 116, 135, 139
CEREBRAL EDEMA	109
Cerebral Ischemia	119

Cerebral Hemorrhage	101, 119
CerebroMacular Degenerations	150
CERVICAL SPINE FRACTURE	109
Chest Compression	111
chewing ability weak	63, 66, 120
chewing automatic movements	63, 68, 91, 101, 120, 130, 131
CHLORINATED HYDROCARBON TOXICITY	108
CHRONIC TRAUMATIC ENCEPHALOPATHY (CTE)	101, 128, 132, 135, 139, 140
clonic muscle movement	63, 86
clothing soiled, ragged / appearance poor	74, 78, 89, 104, 136
CNS DEGENERATIVE DISORDERS	147
CNS STIMULANTS	104
Coarctation of Aorta; hypertensive encephalopathy DELIRIUM	125
coherent thought process	51, 78, 106, 137
collapse, suddenly falling	57 -64
CONCENTRATION	6, 74, 90, 100, 114, 137
conceptual disorganization of thought process	6, 50, 92, 143
CONSCIENTIOUSNESS/ DEPENDABILITY	9
CONFUSION STATE	103
CONSCIENTIOUSNESS/ DEPENDABILITY	93
Convulsions	101, 109, 118
COPD	101, 113, 117
Cranial Nerve I & II Examination	**82 - 88**
Cranial Nerve III Examination	**82 - 88**
Cranial Nerve IV-VIII Examination	**82 - 88**
Cranial Nerve IX-XII Examination	83 - **87**
CRANIO-VERTEBRAL MALFORMATIONS	147
Crescendo Heart Murmur at apex	111
CREUTZFELDT-JACOB SYNDROME	142, 143
CTE (CHRONIC TRAUMATIC ENCEPHALOPATHY)	101, 128, 132, 135, 139, 140
CUSHING'S SYNDROME	112, 117
CXR shows concentric LVH & prominent ascending aorta	107, 113
CYANIDE POISONING	108
DAWSON'S SUBACUTE SCLEROSING PANENCEPHALITIS	150
Delirium	7, 9, 32, 77, **95-135**, 143
delusions	7, 77, 82, 97
Dementia	7, 9, 32, 37; 89-95, **139-152**
Dementia - Jenicke	**37**-38
DEMENTIA WITH PARKINSON'S DISEASE	142
dental condition poor	66
Depression Scale	33
derailment / alusive thought process	7, 68, 75, 91, 92
deterioration of capacities	7, 77, 83, 134
DIABETIC KETOACIDOSIS	117, 122

Dementia - Jenicke	**37**-38
DEMENTIA WITH PARKINSON'S DISEASE	142
dental condition poor	66
Depression Scale	33
derailment / alusive thought process	7, 68, 75, 91, 92
deterioration of capacities	7, 77, 83, 134
DIABETIC KETOACIDOSIS	117, 122
Diagnostic And Statistical Manual of Mental Disorders	5,32, 99, 102, 113, 116, 121, 135
DIFFERENTIATING NEUROCOGNITIVE DISORDERS	**95**
DIAGNOSTICS	27-41
difficulty "reading" other people's emotions	28,29,30
difficulty expressing anger; "bottling-up" anger	28, 29, 30
difficulty expressing emotions	28, 29, 30
difficulty maintaining eye contact	7, 28-31, 89-93, 143
difficulty starting new projects	71, 89, 102, 107
DISORDERS OF AROUSAL	102, **103-108**,
DISORDERS OF ENERGY METABOLISM with Metabolic Acidosis	117, 126, 149
DISORDERS OF METABOLISM	101
DISSEMINATED INTRAVASCULAR COAGULATION	117
DISSOCIATIVE AMNESIA	131
DISSOCIATIVE IDENTITY DISORDER	131
distractible when asked to attend	12, 32, 46
DIZZINESS / abnormal pulse	46, 52, 54, 57, 108 -111
Dizziness Algorithm	56, 58, 59
DIZZINESS on rising from supine	43, 51, 52
Dizziness Questionnaire	**52**
draw-a-clock	78, 116,137, 138
dream trance states	46, 51, 63,104, 138
DRIVE	6, 19, 37,50, 137
Drug Abuse Screening Test	35
DSM-5	5,32, 99, 102, 113, 116, 121, 135
DYSAUTONOMIA; HYPOTENSIVE/ HYPERTENSIVE	118, 125
early systolic ejection click lower LSB & apex	121
ECG prolonged in longest complex; abnormal Holter Monitor	107, 112, 121
ECG shows prolonged QT, inverted T in II, III, avf & V4-6	107, 112,121
Echocardiogram shows abnormal mitral valve movement	107
edginess / anxiety/ "keyed up"	89
EEG 2.5-3 c.p.s. spike-wave pattern	63, 68, 91, 101, 130
EEG atypical spike-wave complexes	63, 68, 91, 101, 130
EEG focal fast / slow waves	63, 68, 91, 101, 130
ELECTROLYTE DISORDERS	95, 101, 117,126, 149
ENCEPHALITIS/ ENCEPHALOPATHY	119
EpiDural Hematoma	109, 119
Epworth Sleepiness Scale	35

ERGOT POISONING	108, 110
EXAMINATIONS	**4, 73 - 95**
EXAMINATIONS -Mood and Affect	7, 31
EXPRESSIVE LANGUAGE	7, 78, 91, 94, 139, 143
eye - blurred disc	84, 125
eye - central scotoma	84
eye - papilledema	68, 84, 120, 123, 125
eye - pupil abnormal	85
eye - retinal absence of venous pulsations	84
eye papillitis (optic neuropathy)	84
eye-contact poor	28, 74, 89, 114, 121
eyes - corneal reflex lost	86
eyes - deviation / deflection of strabismic eye when covered	73, 91
eyes - double vision	43, 66, 108, 109
eyes - inability to move upward/ inward / downward/ outward	43, 74, 91-98, 102
eyes - ptosis (inability to open eyelid)	43, 74, 91-98, 102
eyes - pupil blink reflex lost	43, 74, 91-98, 102
eyes - pupil dilated	68, 84, 85,104
eyes "opsillopsia" / "dancing eyes"	112
face - pain / weakness	87
facial expressions	50, 89, 129
Falling Down	54 - 72
falling limp to floor	63, 150
FALLING/ FAINTING/ DIZZY SPELL CHECKLIST	54 - 72
Familial SUDANOPHILIC LEUKODYSTROPHY	150
feelings / mood	7, 49, 79, 82, 103
Focal Motor PARTIAL (Jacksonian) Seizure	63,101,118, 130, 131
focus / concentration / processing speed / distractibility	7, 67, 80, 85, 123
forehead wrinkle ability lost	86
FRONTAL LOBE ATROPHY	135, 142
Fronto-Temporal-Parietal Lobar Degeneration FTC	135, **138**, 139, 142, 143
FUNCTIONAL CAPACITIES	6,7, 8, 38, 39, 78,93, 95
Functional Impairment Scale	38,39
FUNCTIONALLY IMPAIRED - mentally or physically	8, 38, 39, 93, 95, 99, 143
FUND OF KNOWLEDGE	6, 74, 78, 79
fundoscopic exam abnormal	82, 33
FUTURE PLANS	6, 78
GENERAL - appearance / apparent age/ hygiene	67, 71, 79
GLASGOW COMA SCALE	104
GLUE-SNIFFING (TOLUENE TOXICITY)	101
GLUTARIC ACIDEMIA TYPE II	101
Grand Mal (Major Motor) Seizure	82, 113, 116
GRAVE'S DISEASE - "thyroid storm" DELIRIUM	124
grooming poor	6, 74, 89

HALLERVORDEN SPATZ (Pantothenate Kinase-Associated NCD)	146
hallucinations	6, 51, 57, 92,**104**,130,138, 143
HALLUCINOGENS	104
HARTNUP'S DISEASE	147
has hobbies still; completes tasks holds job/relationship	7, 71
Head Injury Evaluation	61-65, **109**
head-turning automatic movements	53
headache history	53-59
Health History / R.O.S.	41-65
HEART BLOCK	112
HEART FAILURE	112, 117
heart murmur harsh; +/- thrill; pulse pressure < 30	101, 104
HEPATIC ENCEPHALOPATHY	111, 117, 146
HEPATO-CEREBRAL DEGENERATION of Cirrhosis	146
hidden anger towards self & others; holds resentments	28
history of Rheumatic Fever / strep throats / FANA positive	101, 109
HIV ASSOCIATED NCD	136
homicidal thinking	7, 67, 71, 83
hopelessness / suicidal ideation	7, 49, 67, 71, 77, 82
HUNTINGTON'S DISEASE DEMENTIA	136, 146
Hydrocephalus causing DEMENTIA (Inc./Normal Pressure -Occult)	101, 140
HyperAldosteronism Hypertensive encephalopathy DELIRIUM	125
HYPERCALCEMIA Delirium	121
HYPERPARATHYROIDISM Delirium	121
HYPERTENSIVE ENCEPHALOPATHY Delirium	118, 120, 125
HYPOPHOSPHATASIA	121
HYPOPITUITARY Delirium	125
HYPERTHYROID Hypertensive encephalopathy DELIRIUM	112,124,125
Hyperviscosity Syndrome	113
Hypothyroid delirium	124
Immune Disorders (e.g., S.L.E.) causing DEMENTIA	140
IMPULSE / BEHAVIORAL CONTROL	93
Infectious Disorders causing DEMENTIA	119, 140
INTEGRITY	93
INSIGHT - into one's illness	6,74,78,93,137
insight into one's capacities / intentions	6,74,78,93,137
Intermediate Memory Test	70
IRON POISONING	110
JAUNDICE & HYPERAMMONIA - HEPATIC ENCEPHALOPATHY	101
JUDGMENT	6, 12, 32, 78,104,137, 142
Juvenile Infantile CEREBRO-MACULAR NCD (Batten-Mayou-Spiel-)	150
KETOACIDOSIS	101
"keyed-up" behavior	77
knowledge of bordering states	7, 67

knowledge of current events	6, 74, 78
KRABBE DISEASE	148
lack of forethought / planning	7
LACTIC ACIDOSIS	101, 122
LACUNAR STATE CNS -after T.I.A./Stroke	119, 142, 143, 144
Late Infantile Cerebromacular Degeneration (Bielschowsky)	150
Lead Poisoning	110, 123
LEIGH'S DISEASE	148
LEWY BODY DEMENTIA	91, 135, 138, 141, 143
light reflex impaired/ LOST	73, 74, 91, 98,**103**
LIMBIC DISEASE / DISORDERS	90, 91, 95, 96,129-132, 136
linear thought process	, 67, 81,
lip-smacking movements	53, 55
LONG-TERM MEMORY TEST	141
low motivation to perform task if uninterested	28,29
ORGAN FAILURE (hepatic cirrhosis/ renal failure azotemia/dialysis	140
Major and Mild Neurocognitive Disorders	6, 85, 121, 122
Major and Mild Neurocognitive Disorders - Multiple Etiol.	121, 122
Major and Mild Neurocognitive Disorders - Unspecified	121, 122
MAJOR DEPRESSION	8, 114
Major Motor (Grand Mal) Seizure	46,54,57,63,92,108,120,122,126,128,130,131,142,143
MCAD DEFICIENCY - Disorder of Fatty Acid Metabolism	101, 117, 149
MANIA	7, 89, 91, 113, 126
MEMORY - immediate	7,16,32-36,48, 53,69,70,71,77, 80-86,96,113
MEMORY - intermediate	7,70,77,80,81,113
MEMORY - long-term / remote	69,81,85,115,120,123,125,127,136
MENTAL STATUS EXAMINATION - Memory/ abstract thinking, ETC.	**78**
MERCURY (INORGANIC) POISONING	110
METABOLIC ACIDOSIS progressing to DEMENTIA	140, 149
METHANOL TOXICITY (WOOD ALCOHOL)	108
mid-systolic ejection click on heart auscultation	57
MILD COGNITIVE IMPAIRMENT	95
milestones	6, 131, 150
MILK-ALKALI SYNDROME	121
Minor Motor (Petit Mal) Seizure	48-55
Mitral Valve Prolapse / MITRAL STENOSIS	109, 119
MODERATE HEAD INJURY	109
MOOD	6, 31,50, 59,74,78,89,93,107,126,137
motor automatic movements	63,101,118, 130, 131
movements - voluntary / involuntary	6,21,29,48,53,55,58,**63,** 72, 125, 133
MULTIPLE SYSTEM ATROPHY (Shy-Drager Syndrome)	142, 143
MUSHROOM POISONING	109
MYASTHENIA GRAVIS	117

Myoclonic Seizure	63
naming the presidents	76, 78, 90
NAPTHALENE POISONING	108, 110
NARCOTIC POISONING	109
NCD DIFFERENTIAL CHART	95
NCD DIFFERENTIAL TYPES	96
NEOPLASTIC/CNS paraneoplastic Delirium/ Dementia	130
NEPHROTIC SYNDROME -METABOLIC ACIDOSIS	122
NEURAL CREST TUMOR	112
Neurocognitive Questionnaire	27-41
NEUROLEPTIC MALIGNANT SYNDROME	101
Neurological Examination	**82 -89**
NEUROMYELITIS OPTICA (DEVICS) MULTIPLE SCLEROSIS	150
NEURONAL DEGENERATION (Seitelberger)	150
NEUROSYPHILIS; SYSTEMIC	119
NITRITE/ NITRATE POISONING	108
nystagmus (jerking eye-movements) with dizziness	83, 84, 86, 111, 148
OBJECTIVE NEUROLOGIC RATING SCALE	106
OBJECTIVE TOXICITY RATING SCALE	107
OBSTRUCTIVE SLEEP APNEA	119
OPIATES TOXICITY	104
optic disc "choked"	73
ORGANIC PHOSPHATE POISONING	109
ORIENTATION to time, play, person and cir stance (Why here?)	6, 78, 79, 104, 105, 131
overload / multitasking & contradiction causes shut-down	28
panic / fear brief seizures	16, 29, 52
Paraneoplastic Syndrome of Delirium/Dementia	130, 132
PARKINSON'S DISEASE DEMENTIA	136
Partial / Focal Seizure	63,101,118, 130, 131
PCP TOXICITY	109
PELIZAEUS-MERZBACHER DISEASE	148
PERCEPTION	74, 78, 92, 100, 116, 142, 143
PERSISTENCE	7, 71, 85, 123, 125
personality changes noted	6, 24, 37, 66, 120, 139, 143
Petit Mal (Minor Motor) Seizure	63
pharyngeal reflex lost	76
PHEOCHROMOCYTOMA; hypertensive encephalopathy - DELIRIUM	112, 118, 125
PICK'S DISEASE - BEHAVIORAL LOSS OF SOCIAL INHIBITIONS	138
PICKWICK'S SYNDROME -obesity & compromised ventilation	111
picking at clothes automatisms	63, 90, 115, 116,
PLAQUE (Amyloid Beta 40/42 ratio & APOE genotype) TESTS	137
POLYNEUROPATHY/POLYRADICULONEUROPATHY	55
PONTINE STRUCTURAL LESION	109

Post-Concussion Syndrome	101, 139
prefers visually-presented instructions	28, 29
PROGRESSIVE NON-FLUENT APHASIA	138
PROGRESSIVE SUPRANUCLEAR PALSY	142, 143
PRION ASSOCIATED NEROCOGNITIVE DISORDER	135
pseudodementia	7, 129
pseudopapilledema	84
Psychiatric Assessment	74-82
Psychomotor (Temporal Lobe) Seizure	63, 101, 118, 130, 131
PULMONARY HYPOPERFUSION/ EMBOLISM	119
QT segment on ekg PROLONGED	101
reading, writing, speaking	40, 46, 78
RENAL TUBULAR ACIDOSIS	101
retinal pigmentation abnormal	84
rigid adherence to rules & routines	28, 29
Roberts-2 "popular pull" imperception	30, 78, 116
sarcastic / negativistic/ critical	28, 29
SCHILDER'S BALOS SCHOLTZ DIFFUSE SCLEROSIS	150
SCHIZOPHRENIA	7, 89-93, 103, 143
SEDATIVES/HYPNOTICS TOXICITY	104
Seizure Algorithm	59, 63
Seizure History	60-65
self-stimulation to reduce anxiety	28, 29
SEMANTIC FTD	138
SET TEST for categorization lost in Alzheimer's Disease ("FACTS")	137
SEVERE HEAD INJURY	109
showing unusually strong food preferences / aversions	28, 29
SHY-DRAGER SYNDROME MULTIPLE SYSTEM ATROPHY	142, 143
SICKLE-CELL DISEASE; EMBOLISM TO BRAIN	119
SICK SINUS SYNDROME	112, 118
SLEEP DISORDERS	70, 71
SLEEP HISTORY	70
SLEEP/WAKE CYCLE & receptors	96
S.L.E. DEMENTIA with psychosis	152
smell sense is lost	84, 137
SOCIAL COMPETENCE AND/OR TEAMWORK	93
speaking, reading, writing	7, 22, 39, 48, 71
SPEECH & LANGUAGE	6, 91, 102, 104, 105, 106, 114, 120, 137
speed of thought process is rapid	7, 81, 123
speed of thought process is slow	7, 94, 125
SPINOCEREBELLAR DEGENERATIONS	147
STATUS EPILEPTICUS	109
STEEL-RICHARDSON-OLZEWSKI PROGRESSIVE SUPRANUCLEAR	142, 143

stiffening of body "boardlike"	46, 63
STIMULANT DRUG (CNS) TOXICITY	104
STOKES-ADAMS SYNDROME - HEART BLOCK	112
SUBACUTE COMBINED DEGENERATION (SHY-DRAGER)	111, 142
SubArachnoid Hemorrhage	113
SubDural Hematoma	109, 119
suicidal thinking	74, 78, 92, 93, 139
SUNDOWNER SYNDROME	101
SupraVentricular TACHYCARDIA	112
SYDENHAM'S CHOREA	152
SYNCOPE	**56-64**, 112
Systemic Luis Erythematosis	119
TAKAYASU'S ARTERITIS	120
TACHYCARDIA	112
taste ability lost	45, 86, 87
taste sense lost	45, 86, 87
Tensilon Test positive (myasthenia)	87, 111, 117
TESTS for Amyloid Beta 40/42 ratio plaques and APOE genotypes	137
thin, asthenic body habitus with mid-systolic heart murmur	57
Third Degree Heart Block	112
THOUGHT CONTENT	7, 67, 82
Thought Form Checklist for "formal thought disorder"	68
THOUGHT PROCESS	7, 67, 81
THYROTOXICOSIS (THYROID STORM)	112, 117, 124
TOLUENE TOXICITY (GLUE SNIFFING)	101
tongue atrophy or fasciculations	82-88
tongue weak on protrusion or deviation	82-88
tonic-clonic jerking movements	46, 63
TORSADES DE POINTES (QT prolonged)	101
TRANSIENT GLOBAL AMNESIA	130
TRANSIENT ISCHEMIC ATTACK (T.I.A.)	120
TRAUMATIC BRAIN INJURY / CTE	135, 140
uncomfortable competing with others	28, 29
unconsciousness spells	48-63
unrealistic future plans	78, 79
Uremia	101
vacant stare - avoiding eye contact	84, 89
VASCULAR DEMENTIA	135, 139
VERTEBRO-BASILAR ARTERY stenosis	119
VERTEBRO-BASILAR MIGRAINE	120
vertigo / "room spinning around"	57, 85, 86, 108, 110, 120
visual acuity is impaired	43, 57, 66, 82, 83, 86, 92, 108, 109, 110, 120, 125
VITAMIN DEFICIENCY; Subacute Combined Degeneration/ Wernicke	111, 140

VITAMIN DEFICIENCY; Subacute Combined Degeneration/ Wernicke	111, 140
VITAMIN D TOXICITY	101, 121
VON HIPPEL LINDAU DISEASE	147
WILSON'S DISEASE	146
Word-finding ability	94
word-salad thought process	106
work performance	7, 38, 39
writing, speaking, reading	40, 46, 78
YELLOW PHOSPHOROUS POISONING	110

REFERENCES

Adams & Victor's **Principles of Neurology**, 6th Edition, Raymond D. Adams, Maurice Victor, ISBN-13: 978-0070674394

Astra Zeneca Pharmaceuticals LP, **Manual of Rating Scales For the Assessment of Mood Disorder**, 2004, Wilmington, DE 19850-5437.

Diagnosis and Statistical Manual of Mental Disorders, 5th Edition, June 2013, ISBN 978-0-89042-554-1.

2020 Ferri's CLINICAL ADVISOR, Fred F. Ferri, M.D., F.A.C.P., Elsevier Inc. 2020. ISBN 978-0-323-67254-2.